mind

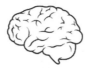

over

medicine

PRAISE FOR *MIND OVER MEDICINE*

"In this elegant and exhaustively researched book Dr. Lissa Rankin offers compelling evidence both that human beings are far more than an assemblage of chemicals and electrical signalling, and that that the mind is the very best drug there is. Prepare to open yourself to an entirely new paradigm of medicine, health, and healing."

— **Lynne McTaggart**, international best-selling author of *The Field, The Intention Experiment,* and *The Bond*

"What a pleasure it is to see the next generation of physicians waking up to what I call real medicine—the kind that acknowledges our true power to heal and be well."

— **Christiane Northrup, M.D.**, OB/GYN physician and author of the *New York Times* bestsellers: *Women's Bodies, Women's Wisdom* and *The Wisdom of Menopause*

"In this book, Lissa Rankin clearly states what many health care providers (not to mention patients) already know: the way our society's physicians are trained, pressured, and overworked is in many ways inimical to the process of healing. In her life, her work, and her words, Dr. Rankin demonstrates a new way to combine the brilliance of modern science with the wisdom of the heart. Anyone who will ever need a doctor, and certainly anyone who will ever be a doctor, will be enriched and enlightened by her ideas. Just reading Mind Over Medicine is a genuinely healing experience."

— **Martha Beck, Ph.D.**, author of *Finding Your Way in a Wild New World*

"Being my own inner physician for years means that I'm SUPER thrilled about Dr. Lissa Rankin's brilliant new book, Mind Over Medicine. She marries intuition with science and shows us all our healing SUPERPOWERS, and how to live our lives this way. And, Lissa's writing style is so exuberant and deep at the same time, it makes me feel like I can do handstands on the ocean!"

— **SARK**, author of 16 books, artist, and founder of PlanetSARK.com

"Mind Over Medicine modernizes age old messages of wisdom and makes them easier to understand and apply to modern day lifestyles. This book contains much wisdom in easy-to-apply lessons we can all learn from."

— **Bernie Siegel, M.D.**, author of *Love, Medicine & Miracles*

"With humor, warmth, and compelling research, Dr. Lissa Rankin's Mind Over Medicine begins to heal the most critical fracture of our time—the break between our mind, bodies, and spirit. When it comes to our physical and emotional health, we need to tap into our own wisdom and find our voices. Lissa's passion and experiences make her the perfect guide for this journey."

— **Brené Brown, Ph.D.**, *New York Times* best-selling author of *Daring Greatly: How the Courage to be Vulnerable Transforms the Way We Live, Love, Parent, and Lead*

mind

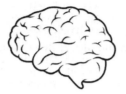

over

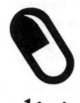

medicine

Scientific Proof You Can Heal Yourself

Dr Lissa Rankin

HAY HOUSE

Carlsbad, California • New York City • London • Sydney
Johannesburg • Vancouver • Hong Kong • New Delhi

First published and distributed in the United Kingdom by:
Hay House UK Ltd, Astley House, 33 Notting Hill Gate, London W11 3JQ
Tel: +44 (0)20 3675 2450; Fax: +44 (0)20 3675 2451
www.hayhouse.co.uk

Published and distributed in the United States of America by:
Hay House Inc., PO Box 5100, Carlsbad, CA 92018-5100
Tel: (1) 760 431 7695 or (800) 654 5126
Fax: (1) 760 431 6948 or (800) 650 5115
www.hayhouse.com

Published and distributed in Australia by:
Hay House Australia Ltd, 18/36 Ralph St, Alexandria NSW 2015
Tel: (61) 2 9669 4299; Fax: (61) 2 9669 4144
www.hayhouse.com.au

Published and distributed in the Republic of South Africa by:
Hay House SA (Pty) Ltd, PO Box 990, Witkoppen 2068
Tel/Fax: (27) 11 467 8904
www.hayhouse.co.za

Published and distributed in India by:
Hay House Publishers India, Muskaan Complex, Plot No.3, B-2,
Vasant Kunj, New Delhi 110 070
Tel: (91) 11 4176 1620; Fax: (91) 11 4176 1630
www.hayhouse.co.in

Distributed in Canada by:
Raincoast, 9050 Shaughnessy St, Vancouver BC V6P 6E5
Tel: (1) 604 323 7100; Fax: (1) 604 323 2600

A catalogue record for this book is available from the British Library.

ISBN: 978-1-84850-960-3

Printed and bound in Great Britain by TJ International, Padstow, Cornwall.

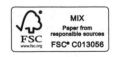

In loving memory of David,
my beloved Daddy,
the original Dr. Rankin

CONTENTS

FOREWORD

With this insightful book, Dr. Lissa Rankin reintroduces us to a wellspring of ancient intelligence that shows the power you have over your own health. She carries the torch passed down to her by some of the greatest mind-body healers of our time. Folks like Bernie Seigel, Dean Ornish, Deepak Chopra, Candace Pert, Jon Kabat-Zinn, and countless other pioneers before her. Quite simply, Lissa is the leading voice of the next generation of medical trailblazers and innovators who marry hard evidence with heart. In the still, quiet place where science meets the miraculous, *Mind Over Medicine* triumphs.

The mind-body connection has been the focus of my writing for more than a decade. As a person ~~living~~ thriving with a chronic disease, I've searched for answers to some of the toughest health questions around, and what I've stumbled on has radically transformed my life. And *Mind Over Medicine* powerfully reinforces what I've learned.

As technology and science continue to make remarkable advances, we have so much at our fingertips, advantages our ancestors never had. And yet, it's common to experience heightened stress and anxiety. Many of us are totally strung out. We're worried about our finances, our relationships, and an uncertain future. We feel separate, afraid, and alone. These feelings and more lead to tangible physical changes in the body.

Contrary to what we previously believed, our genes are not fixed. The study of epigenetics proves that our genes are actually fluid, flexible, and highly influenced by our environment. And here's the best news, just because you have a genetic predisposition for x, y, and z, doesn't mean those genes will actually express themselves. External lifestyle triggers like nutrition, environment, exercise, positive or negative thoughts, and emotions literally affect your DNA. So what truly runs in your family: heart disease and diabetes, or donuts and sausage? How about gratitude and appreciation, or belittlement and abuse? Change your thoughts, change your behaviors. Change your behaviors, change your biochemistry.

As Lissa explains, our minds can make us sick and they can make us well. Our feelings and beliefs impact our every cell. How we speak to ourselves matters. Whether or not we feel and express love affects our well-being. That very notion empowers me. It fills me with hope and curiosity. She explains, using some of the latest scientific research that you have access to, a treasure trove of regenerative information, a pharmacy of sorts, complete with an inner MD who always knows exactly what to prescribe.

With this knowledge, you can choose health. Imagine how good it would feel to truly adore and appreciate the skin you're in. To release the blocks that hold you back and embrace the unique beauty that makes you such a vital part of the human race. Pause for a moment. Picture it. See yourself happy, whole, and at ease. Feel your worth. Feel your strength. Feel your healing potential.

Our thoughts hold more medicine than many of the astonishing breakthroughs of our time, and in this book, Lissa creates a new model for well-being focused on harnessing this power. If you follow her stellar advice, you will not only change your life, you may just save it. If you've forgotten how remarkable you are, *Mind Over Medicine* will guide you home. I know that I've only just begun to scratch the surface of the vast wisdom stored in my miraculous body.

Blessings to you on your journey to health, spiritual wealth, and sustainable happiness.

Kris Carr
New York Times best-selling author, cancer thriver, and wellness activist

INTRODUCTION

"There is no illness of the body apart from the mind."

— SOCRATES

What if I told you that caring for your body is the *least* important part of your health . . . that for you to be truly vital, other factors are more important? What if the key to health isn't just eating a nutritious diet, exercising daily, maintaining a healthy weight, getting eight hours of sleep, taking your vitamins, balancing your hormones, or seeing your doctor for regular checkups?

Certainly, these are all important, even critical, factors to optimizing your health. But what if something else is even more important?

What if you have the power to heal your body just by changing how your mind thinks and feels?

I know it sounds radical, especially coming from a doctor. Trust me, I was just as skeptical when I first discovered the scientific research suggesting that this might be true. Surely, I thought, the health of the human body isn't as simple as thinking ourselves well or worrying ourselves sick.

Or is it?

A few years ago, after 12 years of conventional medical education and 8 years of clinical practice, I had been thoroughly indoctrinated into the dogmatic principles of evidence-based medicine, which I worshipped like the Bible. I refused to trust anything I couldn't prove with a randomized, controlled clinical trial. Plus, having been raised by my father, a very conventional physician who made fun of anything New Age, I was as hard-nosed, closed-minded, and cynical as they come.

The medicine I had been trained to practice didn't support the idea that you can think yourself well or make yourself sick with the power of your thoughts and emotions. Sure, my medical-school professors diagnosed some illnesses that lacked biochemical explanations as "all in the patient's head," but those patients were promptly and quietly referred to psychiatrists, while eyes were rolled and heads were shaken.

It's no wonder the notion that the mind might have the power to heal the body would be threatening to many mainstream doctors. After all, we spend a decade learning the tools that supposedly give us mastery over other people's bodies. We want to believe that the time, money, and energy we've put into becoming doctors isn't wasted. We're professionally and emotionally invested in the idea that if something breaks down physically, you must seek our expertise. As doctors, we like to believe we know your body better than you do. The whole medical establishment is based on such a notion.

Most people are happy to function within this paradigm. The alternative—that you have more power to heal your own body than you've ever imagined—lobs the responsibility for health back into your court, and many people feel like that's just too much responsibility. It's much easier to hand over your power and hope someone smarter, wiser, and more experienced can "fix" you.

But what if we've got it all wrong? What if, by denying the fact that the body is naturally wired to heal itself and the mind operates this self-healing system, we're actually sabotaging ourselves?

As physicians, things inevitably happen on our watch that science simply can't explain. Even the most closed-minded doctors witness patients who get well when, by every scientific rationale, they shouldn't. When we witness such things, we can't help questioning everything we hold dear in modern medicine. We start to wonder if there is something more mystical at play.

Doctors don't usually discuss this possibility in front of patients, but they do whisper about it in the doctors' lounges of hospitals and inside conference rooms at Ivy League universities. If you're curious and you pay attention—like I do—you hear stories, stories that blow your mind.

You hear people whispering about the woman whose cancer shrank away to nothingness during radiation. Only afterward did the doctors discover that the radiation machine was busted. She hadn't actually received one lick of radiation, *but she believed she had.* So did her doctors.

They talk about the woman who had a heart attack followed by bypass surgery, then wound up in shock, which led to full-blown renal failure believed to be fatal without treatment. When the doctors offered dialysis, she refused treatment, not wanting to endure more invasive procedures. For nine days, her kidneys made no urine, but on the tenth day, she started peeing. Two weeks later, with no treatment, she was back to working out and her kidney function was better than before her surgery.

Then there's the man who had a heart attack who refused heart surgery only to have his "incurably" blocked coronary arteries open up after changing his diet, beginning an exercise program, doing yoga, meditating daily, and attending group therapy sessions.

Another patient who was hospitalized in the ICU and whose organs were shutting down from stage 4 lymphoma had a near-death experience, became one with pure, unconditional love, and instantly knew that if she chose not to cross over to the other side, her cancer would disappear almost at once. Less than a month later, her lymph nodes were biopsied and no evidence of cancer remained.

Yet another woman broke her neck. After being taken to a hospital and getting X-rays that confirmed that she had broken her neck in two places, she opted to refuse medical intervention and saw a faith healer instead, despite her doctors' vehement objections. Without any medical treatment, she was out jogging a month later.

One story floating around claims that a research protocol for a chemotherapy drug called EPOH was getting some marginally positive results, but one oncologist was demonstrating wildly successful outcomes. Why? Rumor has it he switched around the name of the drug protocol when he discussed it with patients. Instead of injecting his patients with EPOH, he injected them with HOPE.

Because I write a popular blog and attract a large, committed tribe of remarkable readers from around the globe, I hear things like this all the time. As I began sharing these supposedly true stories with my readers, more hard-to-believe stories flooded into my e-mail inbox. A woman with Lou Gehrig's disease went to see the healer John of God, and afterward her neurologist proclaimed her cured. A paralyzed man made a pilgrimage to the healing waters of Lourdes and left walking. A woman with stage 4 ovarian cancer "just knew" she wasn't going to die, and, after rallying the support of the people who love her, is still alive ten years later. A man with blocked coronary arteries diagnosed after a heart attack was told he would die within a year if he didn't have heart surgery. After refusing surgery, he lived 20 more years and died—not from heart disease—at 92.

As I heard these stories, I couldn't ignore the gnawing voice within me. Surely, these people couldn't all be liars. But if they weren't lying, the only explanation was something *beyond* what I had learned in conventional medicine.

It got me thinking. We know spontaneous, unexplainable remissions sometimes happen. Every doctor has witnessed them. We just shrug our shoulders and go on about our business, usually accompanied by a dull, unnerving sense of dissatisfaction because we can't explain the remission with logic.

But in the back of my mind, I've always pondered whether it's possible we have any control over this process. If the "impossible" happens to one person, is there anything we can learn from what that person did? Are there similarities among the patients who get lucky? Are there ways to optimize the chances of spontaneous remission, especially when effective treatment doesn't exist in the standard medical toolbox? And what, if anything, can doctors do to facilitate this process?

I couldn't help wondering if, perhaps, by not at least *considering* the possibility that patients might have some control over healing themselves, I was being an irresponsible doctor and violating the sacred Hippocratic Oath. Surely, if I were a good doctor, I would be willing to open my mind in service to the patients I cared for.

But inspiring stories bandied about in doctor's lounges or floating around on the Internet simply weren't enough to convince me. A scientist by training and a skeptic by nature, I needed cold, hard proof, and when I started asking for it, I came up short.

I did my best to investigate the rumors I was hearing. I started asking the people telling me their stories to prove them. Could they show me slides under the microscope? Could I talk to the mechanic responsible for the radiation machine? Could I see the medical records?

I was mostly disappointed. When I asked for medical records or studies as backup, most people apologized. "It was so long ago." "There was definitely a study, but I don't have the reference." "My doctor retired, so I can't put you in touch." "They threw away my medical records."

Even the instances of self-healing I vaguely remembered witnessing in the earlier days of my own practice were out of my reach. I hadn't kept notes. I couldn't remember names. I didn't know how to contact these people. I kept hitting dead ends.

Yet the more questions I asked online, the more stories kept flowing in. When I started getting nosy with my physician friends, every doctor I asked told me jaw-dropping stories of unexplained spontaneous healings, patients who wound up cured from "incurable" illnesses, leaving those who pronounced them "terminal" looking like fools. But still, they had no proof.

By this point, I was intrigued, bordering on obsessed. My curiosity led me to dig deeper. After hundreds of e-mails and dozens of interviews, I came to believe that something real was happening to these patients whose stories became lore in metaphysical books and on the Internet. Although it's tempting to dismiss the often ridiculous-sounding stories of patients who claim to have healed themselves, if you're a doctor who cares about helping others heal, you can't ignore what you hear. The more you listen, the more you start to wonder just what the body is capable of.

Most doctors, if you get them away from their often critical and judgmental colleagues, will admit this: deep down, they believe that when it comes to the healing process, some crossover between the mystical and the physiological is at play, and that the common ground that connects the two is the great and powerful mind. But few say so out loud for fear of being labeled quacks.

The mind-body link has been advocated by medical pioneers for decades. Yet, in spite of this, it has failed to shoulder its way into the mainstream medical community. As a young doctor, I received my medical degree well after renowned physicians such as Bernie Siegel, Christiane Northrup, Larry Dossey, Rachel Naomi Remen, and Deepak Chopra had raised awareness about the mind-body link, and you might think their teachings would have been included as part of my medical education. But I was largely unfamiliar with their work until long after I finished medical school. Not until I began doing my own research did I even read their books.

Once I finally did, I was pissed. How did I not know who these open-minded, open-hearted doctors were? And why were their books not required reading for med students and first-year residents?

As I learned more, I got all riled up and that passion turned into a mission that fueled several years' worth of research and writing. I started reading every mind-body medicine book I could find. I also started blogging, tweeting, and posting on Facebook about what I was learning, which only increased the frequency with which I heard stories from people who had experienced what can only be described as medical miracles. I was riveted. The evidence was mounting. But nothing I was hearing counted as "science." I craved scientific proof that it wasn't total nonsense.

So I kept researching, willing my mind to stay open, as I learned more about how the mind could affect the body. Part of me was open to the whole mind-body concept. It made intuitive sense to me. But another part of me was wildly resistant. To believe what I was learning would require letting go of much of what I had been taught, both from my very traditional physician father and from my medical-school teachers.

One of the first books I studied, Harvard professor Anne Harrington's mind-body-medicine history book, *The Cure Within*, left me feeling physically dizzy and viscerally unsettled. In the book, she refers to the mind-body phenomenon as "bodies behaving badly," meaning that sometimes bodies don't respond the way they "should," and the only way we can explain such mysteries is through the power of the mind.[1]

As examples of bodies behaving badly, Harrington tells stories of children living in institutional settings whose material needs were all met but who wound up developmentally and mentally stunted because they were improperly loved. She also cites 200 cases of blindness in a group of Cambodian women forced by the Khmer Rouge to witness the torture and slaughter of their loved ones. Although medical examination could find nothing wrong with the eyes of these women, they claimed to have "cried until they could not see."[2]

Clearly, something was up. The butterflies in my belly drove me to dig deeper, and as I did, I became fascinated with understanding how these things happened. What proof did we have that the power of the mind could transform the body? What physiological forces could explain such occurrences? And what might we do to harness these healing powers?

If I could answer these questions, I could begin to make sense, not just of the mind-boggling stories people were telling me, but of the purpose of my own life and my role as a healer.

At the time I was researching the mind-body link, my place in the world of medicine was unclear to me. After 20 years of medicine, I had become disillusioned with our broken health-care system, which required me to churn through 40 patients a day, often scheduled in hurried seven-and-a-half-minute slots, leaving little time for us to actually talk, much less bond. I almost quit when a longtime patient told me she had planned to confess to a sensitive health issue she was hiding from me. She rehearsed what she would say for days, with the support of her husband. But when it came time for her to spill the beans, apparently, I never removed my hand from the exam-room door. She told me my hair was disheveled and I was dressed in dirty scrubs. She suspected I had been up all night delivering babies—and I probably had been. Although she knew I was probably tired, she kept praying I would touch her arm, sit down on the stool next to her, and offer enough tenderness and connection to make her feel safe to talk about her concern.

But she says my eyes were blank. I was a robot too busy to let go of the door handle.

When I read that letter, I got choked up, felt a hiccup in my chest, and knew in my heart that practicing this kind of medicine was not what drew me to my profession. I had been called to medicine the way some are called to the priesthood, not to churn out rote prescriptions and blow through physical exams like a machine, but to be a healer. What drew me to the practice of medicine was the desire to touch hearts, to hold hands, to offer comfort amid suffering, to enable recovery when possible, and to alleviate loneliness and despair when cure wasn't possible.

If I lost that, I lost everything. Every day of being a doctor was chipping away at my integrity. I knew the kind of medicine my soul wanted to practice, yet I felt helpless to reclaim the doctor-patient connection I craved, as well as victimized by managed-care companies, the pharmaceutical industry, malpractice lawyers, politicians, and other factors that threatened to widen the rift between me and my patients.

I felt like a fraud, a sellout, a cheap, plastic knockoff of the doctor I dreamed of being back when I was an idealistic medical student. But what were my alternatives? I was the sole breadwinner in my family, responsible for covering my medical-school debt, my husband's graduate-school debt, the mortgage, and my newborn daughter's college fund. Quitting my job was out of the question.

Then my dog died, my healthy young brother wound up in full-blown liver failure as a rare side effect of a common antibiotic, and my beloved father passed away from a brain tumor—all in two weeks.

It was the last straw.

With no backup plan or safety net, I left medicine, planning never to look back. Selling the house, liquidating my retirement account, and moving my family to the country to live a simple life, I chalked the whole doctor thing up to one big fat mistake and planned to be a full-time artist and writer.

By that point, I had lost touch with what I was here on this earth to do. I spent a few years blogging, writing books, and making art, yet nothing felt as pressing to me as the calling that had led me to medical school. Something in my soul still yearned to be of service. Painting and writing felt too solitary, too selfish even, as if I was indulging creative endeavors I loved, but at the expense of my calling.

I barely slept for months, and when I did, I dreamed of helping sick patients, of sitting at their bedsides, of listening to their stories with no eye on my watch and no hand on the door. I'd wake up in tears, as if I was mourning a piece of my soul.

In 2009, I began blogging about what I missed about medicine, what I loved about medicine, what originally drew me to the practice of medicine. I wrote about how I consider medicine a spiritual practice, how you practicé medicine, the way you practice yoga or meditation, like you'll never fully master it. I wrote about how the doctor-patient relationship, when treated with the awe it deserves, is sacred, and how I longed to reclaim it. I wrote about how medicine had wounded me, and how, in turn, I had inadvertently wounded others.

Patients and healers of all types started writing me e-mails, telling me their stories, posting comments on my blog, and something in me lit up, something that felt like an opportunity to be of service. The tribe of people I attracted started healing *me*.

Around this time is when those remarkable stories of patients who healed themselves from *incurable* and *terminal* illnesses started trickling in from around the world. In spite of my initial resistance to getting sucked back into the world of medicine, I found myself drawn to the conversations happening on my blog.

I wasn't searching for a way back to medicine. For the first few years, when signs from the Universe began pointing me back to my calling as a healer, I shook my head and hightailed it in the other direction.

But callings are funny that way. You don't get to choose your calling. It chooses you. And while you can quit your job, you can't quit your calling.

One serendipity after another led me down an unplanned, uncharted path, as if birds were dropping crumbs, blazing a trail to my Holy Grail. Books fell off the shelf. Physicians appeared on my path with messages for me. People in my online community sent me articles. Unbidden visions appeared like movies in my mind while I was hiking. Dreams appeared. Teachers called.

I started waking up from the deep anesthesia my medical education and years of practice had induced, and in my groggy haze, I began to see the light. One question led to another, and before I realized what was happening, I was knee-deep in journal articles, trying to ferret out the truth about what was happening in the body when the mind was healthy and why we get sick when the mind is unhealthy. I realized that I didn't have to order lab tests, prescribe drugs, or operate in order to be of service as a doctor. I could help even more people by discovering the truth about how to help people heal themselves.

What followed was a deep dive into the gospels of modern medicine, the peer-reviewed medical literature, where I sought scientific proof that you can heal yourself in journals like the *New England Journal of Medicine* and the *Journal of the American Medical Association*. What I found changed my life forever, and my hope is that it will change your life and the lives of your loved ones.

This book chronicles my journey of discovery and shares with you the scientific data I uncovered, which changed my whole outlook on how medicine should be delivered and received. Once I read this data, I knew I could never again pull the wool back over my eyes.

Is there scientific data to support the seemingly miraculous stories of self-healing that float around? You betcha. There's proof that you can radically alter your body's physiology just by changing your mind. There's also proof that you can make yourself sick when your mind thinks unhealthy thoughts. And it's not just mental. It's physiological. How does it happen? Don't worry. I'll also explain exactly how unhealthy thoughts and feelings translate into disease and how healthy thoughts and feelings help the body repair itself.

But there's more. There's proof that doctors might facilitate your recovery, not so much because of the treatments they prescribe, but because of the authority you ascribe to them. There's also proof that one surprising factor can benefit your health more than eliminating cigarettes, that something you may consider unrelated to the health of the body can add more than seven years to your life, that one fun thing can dramatically reduce the number of doctor visits you'll need, that one positive shift in your mental attitude can make you live ten years longer, that one work habit can increase your risk of dying, and that a pleasurable activity you probably never linked to a healthy life can dramatically reduce your risk of heart disease, stroke, and breast cancer.

These are just a few of the scientifically verifiable facts I share in this book, which have radically changed how I think about medicine.

This book is divided into three parts. In Part One, I'll make the argument that the mind has the power to alter the body physiologically through a potent combination of positive belief and the nurturing care of the right health-care providers. In Part Two, I'll show you how the mind can alter the body's physiology based on the life choices you make, including the relationships you choose to nurture, your sex life, the work you do, your financial choices, how creative you are, whether you're an optimist or a pessimist, how happy you are, and how you spend your leisure time. I'll also teach you one valuable tool you can use anywhere—one that could save your life.

All of this will set you up for Part Three, where I introduce you to a radical new wellness model I've created and guide you through the six steps to healing yourself. By the time you finish the book, you'll have made your own diagnosis, written your own prescription, and created a clear action plan designed to help you make your body ripe for miracles.

Keep in mind that the tips I give you aren't just for sick people, but also for healthy people interested in preventing disease. I don't want you to wait until your body starts screaming at you with life-threatening diseases. Instead, I want to teach you how to listen to the whispers from your body: these are touchstones on your path to optimal health, leading you away from what predisposes you to illness and toward what has been scientifically proven to result in better health and vital longevity.

What I'm about to reveal to you may surprise you, even, perhaps, threaten you. But please, do your body a favor and, as you read this book, try to withhold your judgments, open your mind, and be willing to shift how you think about your body and your health. What I'm about to share with you may challenge long-held beliefs, knock you out of your comfort zone, and make you question whether I'm making this stuff up. But I swear I'm not. Throughout this book, I make every effort to back up what might seem like far-out statements with scientific references.

Because I know that what I'm about to teach you will raise eyebrows, I've written this book just for the people who are skeptical, as I was. I've laid out the book to walk you through my argument as if a jury of my physician peers were judging me. But it's not so much the doctors I'm aiming to convince. Sure, I hope they listen, because if they do, the face of modern medicine as we know it will change forever.

But really, I'm writing this book for *you*—for every person who has ever been sick, anyone who has ever loved someone with an illness, and anyone who wants to prevent illness. You're the one I yearn to help, because in my heart, I long to end suffering and help you optimize the chance that you will live a long, vital, healthy life. That mission is what called me to medicine in the first place.

As you read, I ask only that you stay with me. Give me a chance to expand your mind the way mine has been blown open. Let me help you heal your thoughts so your body can follow. And give yourself permission to release outdated notions about health and medicine. The future of medicine is upon us. Come, take my hand. Let's explore.

PART ONE

BELIEVE
YOURSELF
WELL

Chapter 1

THE SHOCKING TRUTH
ABOUT YOUR HEALTH BELIEFS

"What we are today comes from our thoughts of yesterday,

and our present thoughts build our life of tomorrow:

our life is the creation of our mind."

— THE DHAMMAPADA

A 1957 case study by Dr. Bruno Klopfer (who famously pioneered the Rorschach inkblot test) reports the story of Dr. Philip West and his patient Mr. Wright. Dr. West was treating Mr. Wright, who had an advanced cancer called lymphosarcoma. All treatments had failed, and time was running out. Mr. Wright's neck, chest, abdomen, armpits, and groin were filled with tumors the size of oranges, his spleen and liver were enlarged, and his cancer was causing his chest to fill up with two quarts of milky fluid every day, which had to be drained in order for him to breathe. Dr. West didn't expect him to last a week.

But Mr. Wright desperately wanted to live, and he hung his hope on a promising new drug called Krebiozen. He begged his doctor to treat him with the new drug, but the drug was only being offered in clinical trials to people who were believed to have at least three months left to live. Mr. Wright was too sick to qualify.

But Mr. Wright didn't give up. Knowing the drug existed and believing the drug would be his miracle cure, he pestered his doc until Dr. West reluctantly gave in and injected him with Krebiozen. Dr. West performed the procedure on a Friday, but deep down, he didn't believe Mr. Wright would last the weekend.

To his utter shock, the following Monday, Dr. West found his patient walking around out of bed. According to Dr. Klopfer, Mr. Wright's "tumor masses had melted like snowballs on a hot stove" and were half their original size. Ten days after the first dose of Krebiozen, Mr. Wright left the hospital, apparently cancer-free.

Mr. Wright was rockin' and rollin', praising Krebiozen as a miracle drug for two months until the scientific literature began reporting that Krebiozen didn't seem to be effective. Mr. Wright, who trusted what he read in the literature, fell into a deep depression, and his cancer came back.

This time, Dr. West, who genuinely wanted to help save his patient, decided to get sneaky. He told Mr. Wright that some of the initial supplies of the drug had deteriorated during shipping, making them less effective, but that he had scored a new batch of highly concentrated, ultra-pure Krebiozen, which he could give him. (Of course, this was a bald-faced lie.)

Dr. West then injected Mr. Wright with distilled water.

And a seemingly miraculous thing happened—*again*. The tumors melted away, the fluid in his chest disappeared, and Mr. Wright was feeling great again for another two months.

Then the American Medical Association blew it by announcing that a nationwide study of Krebiozen proved that the drug was utterly worthless. This time, Mr. Wright lost all faith in his treatment. His cancer came right back, and he died two days later.[1]

When I read this, I thought, *Yeah, right.* Surely, this case study couldn't be true. How could cancerous tumors just "melt like snowballs" in response to an injection of water? If the case report was true and something so simple could make a cancer go away, why weren't oncologists wandering through the wards, injecting stage 4 cancer patients with water? If they had nothing to lose, what was the harm?

The whole thing seemed improbable, so I kept looking. Surely, if there was any truth to such a story, there would be similar case studies reported in the literature.

Another patient reported in the *Journal of Clinical Investigation* suffered from severe nausea and vomiting. Instruments measured the contractions in her stomach, indicating a chaotic pattern that matched her diagnosis. Then she was offered a new, magical, extremely potent drug, which her doctors promised would undoubtedly cure her nausea.

Within a few minutes, her nausea vanished, and the instruments measured a normal pattern. But the doctors had lied. Instead of receiving a potent new drug, she had been dosed with ipecac, a substance known not to prevent nausea, but to induce it.

When this nauseated patient believed her symptoms would resolve, her nausea and abnormal stomach contractions disappeared, even when the ipecac should have made them worse.[2]

I sat there, scratching my head. Curious, but it didn't prove anything.

The Healing Power of Fake Surgery

Soon after, I stumbled across an article in the *New England Journal of Medicine* that featured Dr. Bruce Moseley, an orthopedic surgeon renowned for the surgeries he performed on people with debilitating knee pain. To prove how effective his knee surgery was, he designed a brilliantly controlled study.

The patients in one group of the study got Dr. Moseley's famous surgery. The other group of patients underwent an elaborately crafted sham surgery, during which the patient was sedated, three incisions were made in the same location as in the real surgery, and the patient was shown a prerecorded tape of someone else's surgery on the video monitor. Dr. Moseley even splashed water around to mimic the sound of the lavage procedure. Then he sewed the knee back up.

As expected, one-third of the patients getting the real surgery experienced resolution of their knee pain. But what really shocked the researchers was that those getting the sham surgery had the same result! In fact, at one point in the study, those getting the sham surgery were actually having less knee pain than those getting the real surgery, probably because they hadn't undergone the trauma of the surgery.[3]

What did Dr. Moseley's patients think about the study results? As one World War II veteran who benefited from Dr. Moseley's placebo knee surgery said, "The surgery was two years ago and the knee has never bothered me since. It's just like my other knee now."[4]

This study hit me in the gut.

Mr. Wright and the lady getting ipecac were just case studies, and case studies, well known to have biases, aren't considered the gold standard when it comes to interpreting the medical literature. The gold standard by which I was taught to investigate scientific data is the randomized, double-blind, placebo-controlled clinical trial, published in a peer-reviewed journal.

Dr. Moseley's study, a randomized, double-blinded, placebo-controlled clinical trial—published in one of the most highly respected medical journals in the whole world—showed that a significant percentage of patients experienced resolution of their knee pain solely because they *believed* they got surgery.

That was the first real evidence I collected that proved to me that a belief—something that happens solely in the mind—could alleviate a real, concrete symptom in the body. Dr. Moseley's study is what led me to research the placebo effect, the mysterious, powerful, reliably reproducible treatment effect some patients experience when given fake treatment as part of a clinical trial.

The Powerful Placebo

Like every scientist, I had long known about the placebo effect. Fake treatments, such as sugar pills, saline injections, and sham surgeries, are routinely used in modern clinical trials to determine whether a particular drug, surgery, or treatment is truly effective. The term *placebo*, from the Latin for "I shall please," showed up in medical lingo ages ago to indicate inert treatments, traditionally given to neurotic patients to placate them.

For centuries, doctors prescribed treatments without any clinical data to prove that the treatments themselves actually worked. Nobody questioned the treatments the doctor prescribed, and nobody did studies to prove whether something was effective. The doctors simply mixed up tonics, dosed up their patients, and the patients got better, at least a percentage of the time. Or the doctor cut someone open, performed a surgery, and the symptoms improved, or they didn't.

It wasn't until late in the 19th century that the idea of using placebos in clinical research began to emerge. Then, in 1955, the *Journal of the American Medical Association* published a seminal article by Dr. Henry Beecher called "The Powerful Placebo," which made the case that if you dosed people up with drugs, many got better. But if you gave them plain salt water or some other inert ingredient, about a third of them were also cured, not only in their minds, but in real, physiological ways that could be demonstrated in the body.[5]

Suddenly, the concept of "the placebo effect" became a mainstay of contemporary medicine and modern clinical trials were born. Now, good scientific studies bear the burden of proving that the healing effect of the drug or surgery being tested transcends the potent healing power of the placebo. If a drug or surgery demonstrates that it's more effective than a placebo, then it is deemed "effective." If not, the FDA probably won't approve the drug, the surgery will fall out of favor, and the treatment will be dismissed as ineffective, as Dr. Moseley's surgery was. Prescribing treatments that prove to be no better than a placebo is believed to violate the principles of evidence-based medicine. It's what separates the real doctors from the quacks.

Or so I was taught.

It got me thinking. What exactly is the placebo effect? Until I began my research, I had never really stopped to think about it. We all know people in clinical trials get better when you treat them with nothing but a sugar pill. But why?

That's when I realized I had hit the mother lode in my quest for proof that the mind can affect the body. If a percentage of people in clinical trials get better simply because they *believe* they're getting a real drug or surgery, the response they are getting is triggered *solely by the mind*. This realization threw me into a bit of a tailspin.

Evidence That Positive Belief Can Alleviate Symptoms

Back to the medical journals I went, in search of more evidence that the mind's belief that the body is getting a drug or surgery is enough to result in real, live symptom relief. I found that nearly half of asthma patients get symptom relief from a fake inhaler or sham acupuncture.[6] Approximately 40 percent of people with headaches get relief when given a placebo.[7] Half of people with colitis feel better after placebo treatment.[8] More than half of patients studied for ulcer pain have resolution of their pain when given a placebo.[9] Sham acupuncture cuts hot flashes almost in half (real acupuncture helps only a quarter of patients). As many as 40 percent of infertility patients get pregnant while taking placebo "fertility drugs."[10]

In fact, when compared to morphine, placebos are almost equally effective at treating pain.[11] And multiple studies demonstrate that almost all of the happy-making responses patients experience as a result of antidepressants can be attributed to the placebo effect.[12]

It's not just pills and injections that work wonders when it comes to symptom relief. As proven by Dr. Moseley's knee-surgery study, sham surgeries can be even more effective. In the past, ligation of the internal mammary artery in the chest was considered standard treatment for angina. The thought was that, if you blocked blood flow through that artery, you'd shunt more blood to the heart and relieve the symptoms people experience when they're not getting enough coronary blood flow. Surgeons performed this procedure for decades, and almost all the patients experienced improvement in their symptoms.

But were they really responding to the ligation of the internal mammary artery? Or were their bodies responding to the belief that the surgery would be helpful?

On a quest to find out the answer, one study compared angina patients who got their internal mammary arteries ligated with patients who underwent a surgical procedure during which an incision was made on the chest wall, but the artery itself was not ligated.

What happened? Seventy-one percent of those subjected to the sham surgery got better, whereas only 67 percent of those who got the real surgery improved.[13] Internal mammary artery ligation now exists only in medical history.

The data I was collecting was impressive, and I had to wonder if it might be even more impressive if every effort weren't made to minimize the placebo effect in clinical trials. If researchers perceived the placebo effect as a positive phenomenon, something to embrace, perhaps we'd see even higher percentages. But that's not the focus most researchers have. On the contrary, clinical-trial coordinators and medical researchers (who are mostly employed by pharmaceutical companies) go out of their way to diminish the placebo effect. After all, patients who get better from placebos interfere with a drug's ability to get approved for market. To screen out those considered to have "excessive placebo responses," many randomized, double-blinded, placebo-controlled trials of drugs are actually preceded by a "washout phase," in which all participants take an inert pill and anyone who reacts favorably to it is eliminated from the study.

So, if the majority of researchers for new pharmaceuticals weren't in bed with Big Pharma, we might see placebo response rates shoot even higher in clinical trials.

Does Everyone Respond to Placebos?

As I pondered the placebo effect, I found myself doubting whether I would ever respond to a placebo if I were a patient in a clinical trial. After all, I'm a doctor. I've been an investigator in clinical trials myself. I'm a smart cookie, and I think I'd just *know* whether I was getting a real treatment or not. If I suspected I was getting a placebo, clearly it wouldn't help me, right?

It got me thinking. Are certain types of patients more susceptible to placebo responses than others? Is there any data to suggest whether there's a classic profile for placebo responders? Are there personality traits or intelligence measures that predict who gets better when given a sugar pill? Do people with high IQs demonstrate less responsiveness to placebos? Are some people just more gullible?

Turns out scientists have studied this. Researchers originally postulated that those who responded to placebos would have lower IQs or be more "neurotic." But what they discovered is that nearly everybody can be induced to respond to a placebo under the right conditions. We are all susceptible, even doctors and scientists. In fact, some studies suggest that those with higher IQs are even more placebo-responsive.

I took this as good news, because if it's true that the mind's positive beliefs can heal the body, everyone has an equal chance of benefiting from this phenomenon. It's not just gullible people who can believe themselves well; it's smarty-pants people like *you*.

Is Healing from Placebos All in Your Mind?

As my research continued, I couldn't quite wrap my brain around what I was learning. Clearly, the evidence I was collecting looked promising. When patients—not just the gullible ones, but all patients—believe they'll get well, a hearty percentage of them experience clinical improvement.

But this failed to fully satisfy my curiosity. I could make the argument that symptom relief really is all in your head. What is pain, after all, if not a perception in the mind? What is depression, if not a mental state? Even with more tangible diseases like asthma or colitis, maybe you just *perceive* that you can breathe better or *think* you have fewer gastrointestinal symptoms. Maybe the mental perception is changing, but the *body* isn't actually responding in any measurable physiological way. Maybe you just *think* it is, and that's enough to make you feel better.

If it's true that the mind can heal the body, there must be some way to demonstrate that the body is responding, not just with symptom relief, but in physiological ways that can be studied. The next phase of my research led me in search of proof that it's not all in your head, that the mind's belief can actually alter the body's physiology.

With hundreds of thousands of placebo-controlled trials published out there, finding an answer was no small feat, mostly because many of the studies I encountered evaluated symptoms such as headaches, back pain, depression, and decreased libido—which are difficult to quantify. When patients experience relief from such symptoms, it's largely subjective. There's no objective measurement that can prove that what they report is true.

But I did finally find proof that, at least a percentage of the time, real physiological changes happen in the body in response to placebos. When given placebos, bald men grow hair, blood pressure drops, warts disappear, ulcers heal, stomach acid levels decrease, colon inflammation decreases, cholesterol levels drop, jaw muscles relax and swelling goes down after dental procedures, brain dopamine levels increase in patients with Parkinson's disease, white blood cell activity increases, and the brains of people who experience pain relief light up on imaging studies.[14]

These findings convinced me. Placebos don't just change how you feel, they change your biochemistry. This is where things really start to get interesting.

The biochemical impact of the placebo effect potentially throws our whole model of disease into question. But before I made any giant leaps, I wanted to investigate whether there might be other explanations for why people's bodies were responding with both symptom relief and measurable physiological change when treated with placebos. Was it really just positive belief making all those changes in the body, or were there other factors influencing the patients' outcomes? The next phase of my inquiry led me to a few theories.

Five Explanations for the Placebo Effect

When clinical researchers talk about the placebo effect, they're actually referring to a whole host of events that happen when you bring people into a clinical setting, offer them a treatment that they know may be either the treatment under investigation or a placebo, and pay attention to them over a designated period of time. Let's clarify what those five explanations are so we're all using the right lingo.

The most obvious explanation—and the one we would like to believe—is that patients experience symptom relief and manifest physiological change because they think they will. Because of the ethics of informed consent, patients know they may be receiving a placebo, but many patients in a placebo group *believe* they are getting the real treatment when they're not, so they *expect* to get well. In other words, the belief that you will feel differently leads you to feel differently.[15]

But positive belief may not be the only factor contributing to the body's response. The second explanation for why people may get better is classical conditioning. We all know Pavlov's classic dog experiment. Not only did Pavlov's dog salivate in response to his Scooby snack, he also started salivating when he heard the bell that accompanied it. The placebo effect may work in much the same way. If you're used to getting a real drug from a person in a white coat and subsequently getting better, then you may be conditioned to feel better by simply receiving a sugar pill from someone in a white coat.[16] Of course, if this plays a role, it still supports the idea that the mind can heal the body, since classical conditioning demonstrates a clear mind-body link.

The third explanation is that patients participating in clinical trials receive emotional support. Harvard professor Ted Kaptchuk, who studies the placebo effect, often makes the argument in journal articles and in media interviews that the nurturing care of a respected authority figure may account for as much of the placebo effect as positive belief, or even more. A patient in a clinical trial receives attention, support, and sometimes even healing touch, often delivered by an authority figure in a white coat, which has historically come to represent health and healing. We all want to feel seen, heard, even loved, and this alone may relieve symptoms and stimulate positive physiological change, again because of a mind-body link.

The fourth explanation for why people respond to placebos is that, while most studies try to screen out patients who are self-prescribing other treatments, a percentage of patients in clinical trials may still be surreptitiously seeking other treatments that may confound the data. If someone gets better while in a placebo group, it's possible that the other treatment he or she has been sneaking under the table is responsible for the improvement.

The fifth and last explanation is that some patients may get better because the disease resolves itself on its own. After all, the body is a self-healing organism, constantly striving to return to homeostasis. So even if you stuck patients in a dark room, with no treatment or personal attention, a certain percentage of them might improve. Though there is controversy around this subject, a few scientists believe that the phenomenon of spontaneous remission is the only explanation for the placebo effect. Dr. Asbjørn Hróbjartsson and Dr. Peter Gøtzsche's *New England Journal of Medicine* article "Is the Placebo Powerless?" claims that we can't demonstrate a clear placebo effect unless studies also include a no-treatment group that gets neither the drug nor the sugar pill (which most don't).[17] In their study, they found little evidence of any meaningful placebo effect when no-treatment groups were studied, suggesting that it's not positive belief or nurturing care responsible for disease remission, but rather the natural history of the disease.[18] Others criticize this study, however, for its design flaws, claiming that comparing placebo groups from vastly different types of studies, evaluating completely different illnesses, is comparing apples and oranges, making the combined data potentially misleading to interpret.[19]

Regardless, spontaneous remissions can definitely fudge up clinical studies—and they do happen even in the absence of placebos. But doesn't that even more powerfully support the argument that the body is hardwired for self-repair? If even those in no-treatment groups get well a good percentage of the time, doesn't that prove that the body knows how to heal itself? Even if we argued, just for kicks, that the placebo effect doesn't really exist (most experts believe it does), we still know that unexplained spontaneous remissions occur, probably more frequently than we realize, since those who heal themselves outside of a clinical trial aren't tracked by standard health-care systems.

We're left to conclude that although physiological changes experienced with placebos may not be the result of positive belief alone, the placebo effect nonetheless confirms a mind-body link and the body's innate capacity for self-repair.

The Physiology of the Placebo Effect

We know that the placebo effect works. But what are the physiological mechanisms that explain how thoughts, feelings, and beliefs may translate into physiological change?

Researchers argue over the answer to this question, but several theories have been postulated. Thinking positively about getting well may stimulate natural endorphins, which help ameliorate symptoms, relieve pain, and lift your mood. The reverse is also true: when patients who responded positively to placebo were given the opioid blocker naloxone, which blocks natural endorphins, the placebo suddenly stopped being effective.[20]

Believing you'll get better and being nurtured by caring clinical researchers may also relieve physiological stress, known to predispose the body to illness, and initiate physiological relaxation, which is necessary for the body's self-repair mechanisms to operate properly. As first described by Harvard professor Dr. Walter Cannon, the body is equipped with what Cannon named the stress response, also known as the fight-or-flight response, a survival mechanism that gets flipped on when your brain perceives a threat. When this hormonal cascade is triggered by a thought or emotion in the mind, such as fear, the hypothalamic-pituitary-adrenocortical (HPA) axis activates, thereby stimulating the sympathetic nervous system to race into overdrive, pumping up the body's cortisol and adrenaline levels. Over time, filling the body with these stress hormones can manifest as physical symptoms, predisposing the body to disease over time.

But as we'll discuss in more detail in Chapter 8, just as the stress response exists as a survival mechanism designed to help us stay alive in emergency situations, the body also has a counterbalancing relaxation response. When the relaxation response is elicited, stress hormones drop, health-inducing relaxation hormones that counter the stress hormones are released, the parasympathetic nervous system takes over, and the body returns to homeostasis. Only in this rested, relaxed state can the body repair itself. Anything that reduces stress and elicits a relaxation response not only alleviates the symptoms the stress response can cause, but frees the body to do what it does naturally—heal itself.

Positive belief and nurturing care may also alter the immune system. People treated with placebos may experience boosts in immune function which result from flipping off the stress response and initiating the relaxation response. Placebos may also suppress the immune system. In one study, rats were given the immunosuppressive drug cyclophosphamide (mixed with saccharin water). Then the drug itself was removed and the rats were fed only the saccharin water (a placebo). Lo and behold: their immune systems stayed objectively suppressed, even when they were no longer getting the drug, suggesting that even rats may respond to positive belief and nurturing care with measurable physiological immune responses.[21]

Positive belief and nurturing care may also decrease the body's acute phase response, a type of inflammatory response that leads to pain, swelling, fever, lethargy, apathy, and loss of appetite.[22]

The mind-body link may also be mediated by executive functions of the prefrontal cortex of the brain. The fact that placebo responses are disrupted in people with Alzheimer's disease supports this theory.[23] Many with Alzheimer's disease fail to respond to placebos, supporting the idea that an area of the brain related to belief, which may be damaged in a neurological disease state, affects whether a patient responds to placebos. Evolutionary biologist Robert Trivers says that what the brain expects to happen in the near future affects its physiological state. Trivers suggests that those with Alzheimer's don't experience a placebo effect because they are unable to anticipate the future, so their minds cannot physiologically prepare for it.

Placebo responsiveness also correlates to activation of dopamine in the nucleus accumbens, a region of the brain involved in reward mechanisms. Scientists studied the brains of people after they were given money to see how much dopamine they released in the nucleus accumbens. The more the nucleus accumbens responded to a monetary reward, the more likely those patients were to get well with a placebo.[24]

Whatever the mechanism, it's clear that the mind and body communicate through hormones and neurotransmitters that originate in the brain and then leave the brain to signal other parts of the body. So it should come as no surprise to us that what we think and how we feel can translate into physiological changes in the rest of the body.

But it kinda does, doesn't it? We don't talk much about how our thoughts and feelings affect the health of the body. Yet, if they do, why are we not more careful about what we put into our minds? But I'm getting ahead of myself. We'll talk more about how to keep your mind and body healthy in Part Two of this book.

Are All Diseases Equally Placebo-Responsive?

The next question that arose in my quest to understand the placebo effect was whether placebos work for every disease. Do all symptoms and diseases respond to placebos, or are there only certain types of diseases that respond?

What I found is that nearly every clinical trial demonstrates a placebo effect, but some health conditions appear to be more placebo-responsive than others. Placebos seem to be most effective when given to patients with immune-system conditions such as allergies, endocrine disorders such as diabetes, inflammatory conditions such as colitis, mental-health conditions such as anxiety and depression, nervous-system disorders such as Parkinson's and insomnia, cardiac symptoms such as angina, respiratory conditions such as asthma and cough, and, most effectively, pain disorders.

But do placebos work to treat cancer? Heart attacks? Strokes? Liver failure? Kidney disease?

In my research, I couldn't find much data to answer this question, perhaps because treating conditions like these in a clinical trial with a placebo would be considered unethical. With these kinds of life-threatening conditions, new treatments are usually studied against gold-standard treatments that already exist and have been proven to have at least some efficacy. So it's hard to know the limits of what will and won't respond to a placebo.

As I did my research, I got a deep gut feeling that the placebo effect was just the tip of a huge, submerged mind-body iceberg. It got me wandering down mental pathways with questions we may never be able to answer. For example, if patients in clinical trials, who have been informed that they may be treated with placebos, respond with some-times dramatic results, what would happen if we lied to them? What if we created an unethical study that assured everyone they were getting the most effective new drug on the market—and then we gave them placebo treatment? Of course, institutional review boards would never allow such a study because of the principle of informed consent, which protects the rights of patients to know the truth. But what if we could? I suspect the results would knock our socks off. Why? Because, like Mr. Wright with his Krebiozen, there's something powerful that gets set in motion when we believe, without a doubt, that we will get well and are supported by clinicians who share our optimism.

We may never know, but I was coming to believe that the placebo effect was only the beginning. I couldn't help taking a mental leap past the placebo effect to ask myself the bigger, more important question, the elephant in the room we can't help sniffing.

Can we really heal ourselves?

Unlocking the Mystery of Spontaneous Remission

I found part of my answer at a holiday cocktail party at the Institute of Noetic Sciences (IONS) in Petaluma, California, where I was sipping a glass of wine and chatting about my research with IONS president Marilyn Schlitz. When I told her my conundrum, Marilyn smiled at me with a look that said, "No problem!" and referred me to an online data-base that Caryle Hirshberg and Brendan O'Regan had compiled called the Spontaneous Remission Project. This database includes an impres-sive annotated bibliography of 3,500 references from more than 800 journals in 20 different languages, documenting cases of unexplainable spontaneous disease remission. They defined spontaneous remission as "the disappearance, complete or incomplete, of a disease or cancer with-out medical treatment or treatment that is considered inadequate to produce the resulting disappearance of disease symptoms or tumor."[25]

The bibliography includes some astonishing cases. An HIV-positive patient became HIV-negative. One woman with untreated metastatic breast cancer had breast, lung, and femur tumors that resolved spontaneously. The plaques blocking a man's coronary arteries disappeared without treatment. A man's brain aneurysm disappeared. A man with a gunshot wound in the brain recovered with no treatment. A woman with cardiomyopathy in heart failure got better. A woman with thyroid disease experienced a spontaneous cure.[26]

I also became aware of two similarly titled books written in the 1960s, Boyd's *The Spontaneous Regression of Cancer* and Everson and Cole's *Spontaneous Regression of Cancer,* which spawned an increase in the number of such case studies reported in the medical literature.

As I read through case study after case study of spontaneous disease remission, I felt my heart race with excitement. For the most part, the case studies didn't address *how* the spontaneous remissions happened. The patients weren't interviewed about whether they believed they would get well or whether they did anything else remarkable to heal themselves.

But they did give me proof that almost no disease can be called "incurable." Many of the health conditions from which patients spontaneously got well were the kinds of illnesses I was taught were terminal and untreatable. Clearly, I had been taught wrong.

My brain was spinning. I got so many butterflies in my stomach I could barely eat. I lost ten pounds in a few weeks. By this point, I was a converted woman on a mission. ❧

Without a shadow of a doubt, I had proven to myself that the mind can heal the body. I even had a logical physiological explanation for how it happens. But I knew I was only just beginning to understand the complexities of the mind-body link, and I still didn't understand how to harness the mind's power in order to help people prevent illness and treat disease. So I dug deeper.

Chapter 2

THE SUREFIRE WAY TO MAKE YOURSELF SICK AND PREVENT DISEASE REMISSION

"Never affirm or repeat about your health what

you do not wish to be true."

— RALPH WALDO TRINE

After learning so much about the benefits of the placebo effect, I became curious about whether the opposite was also true. If positive beliefs combined with the nurturing care of a clinician can heal the body, does that mean negative beliefs and harsh care from an insensitive clinician can harm the body?

I first wanted to examine the role of negative belief on the body's physiology. Do people have the power to think themselves sick?

Turns out they do. Researchers in San Diego examined the death records of almost 30,000 Chinese-Americans and compared them to over 400,000 randomly selected white people. What they found was that Chinese-Americans, but not whites, die significantly earlier than normal (by as much as five years) if they have a combination of disease and birth year that Chinese astrology and Chinese medicine consider ill-fated. The researchers found that the more strongly the Chinese-Americans attached to traditional Chinese traditions, the earlier they died. When they examined the data, they concluded that the reduction in life expectancy could not be explained by genetic factors, the lifestyle choices or behavior of the patient, the skill of the doctor, or any other variable.

Why did the Chinese-Americans die younger? The researchers concluded that they died younger not because they had Chinese genes, but because they had Chinese beliefs. They believed they would die younger because the stars had hexed them. And their negative belief manifested as a shorter life.[1]

More studies suggest that negative beliefs affect your health. One study showed that 79 percent of medical students report developing symptoms suggestive of the illnesses they are studying.[2] Because they get paranoid and think they'll get sick, they do.

I know this from personal experience. I was a first-year medical student, studying the numerous ways the body can run amuck, burning the midnight oil to memorize the litany of pathological processes that can lead to thousands of different illnesses—everything from porphyria to dengue fever to osteogenesis imperfecta to narcolepsy.

Then suddenly I felt something crawling under my skin. I figured it must be a guinea worm, creeping into my subcutaneous space, ready to break through the skin at any moment and poke its little head out. I also noticed that my feet felt numb when I first woke up in the morning. I was 100 percent certain it was leprosy. The palms of my hands had a speckled pattern that couldn't be anything but fifth disease. And the night sweats, which left me with soaking wet pajamas, could only mean one thing: malaria.

I wound up with multiple chronic health conditions that were diagnosed during my medical education, as I'll explain in detail in Chapter 9, and I strongly suspect my negative beliefs about my health had something to do with it.

I wasn't the only medical student who was afflicted with a whole host of physical symptoms. In fact, the student health clinic didn't seem the least bit surprised to see me and my fellow students, traipsing through just before finals with bizarre complaints and a slew of self-diagnoses. Not only had the doctors and nurses staffing these clinics heard similar complaints from years of experience caring for medical students, they also informed me that the syndrome had actually been given a name: "medstudentitis," or, more formally, "medical student disease."

Think Sick, Be Sick

Whether you're a Chinese-American, a medical student, or *you*, focusing your attention on illness has been scientifically proven to make you sick. Excessive knowledge about what can go wrong with the body can actually harm you. The more you focus on the infinite ways in which the body can break down, the more likely you are to experience physical symptoms.

Scientists call this phenomenon the nocebo effect. While the placebo effect demonstrates the power of positive thinking, expectation, hope, and nurturing care, the nocebo effect demonstrates the power of negative belief. While a placebo was traditionally prescribed to help the patient feel better, the term *nocebo* (Latin for "I shall harm") was introduced to differentiate the pleasing effects of placebos from the harmful effects inert treatments can induce.

For example, if you tell patients in a clinical trial they will be given a pill that will relieve their pain, there's a good chance the pain will go away, even if they're given only a sugar pill. But if you warn them that the treatment might cause nausea and vomiting, there's a high likelihood they'll puke, even when they never got the real drug.

In *Love, Medicine & Miracles*, Dr. Bernie Siegel cites one study showing that patients in a control group for a new chemotherapy drug were given nothing but saline, yet they were warned it could be chemotherapy, and 30 percent of them lost their hair.[3] In another study, hospitalized patients were given sugar water and told it would make them throw up. Eighty percent of them vomited.[4]

Another study examined asthmatics who inhaled a harmless saline solution after being told it contained irritating allergens. Not only did they wheeze and feel short of breath, their bronchi actually constricted. Those who experienced full-blown asthma attacks found relief when they were dosed with the same inert solution and told it would help them.[5]

In one study, more than three-quarters of those who thought they were getting an antihistamine but were actually getting a placebo got drowsy.[6] When study participants were told that the anesthetic nitrous oxide—which normally relieves pain—would cause pain, it did.[7]

In a study published in the *Pavlovian Journal of Biological Sciences,* 34 college students were hooked up to monitors and told that an electric current would be passed through their heads. Study participants were warned that they might experience a headache as a side effect. Although not one volt of current was actually used, more than two-thirds of the students reported headaches.[8]

Even thoughts about death seem to play out. According to Dr. Herbert Benson, a Harvard professor and the president of Mind/Body Medical Institute in Boston, "Surgeons are wary of people who are convinced that they will die. There are examples of studies done on people undergoing surgery who almost want to die to re-contact a loved one. Close to 100 percent of people under those circumstances die."[9]

Patients about to undergo surgery who were "convinced" of their impending death were compared to another group of patients who were merely "unusually apprehensive" about death. While the apprehensive bunch fared pretty well, those who were convinced they were going to die usually did. Similarly, women who believed they were prone to heart disease were four times more likely to die. It's not because these women had poorer diets, higher blood pressure, higher cholesterol, or stronger family histories than the women who didn't get heart disease. The only difference between the two groups was their beliefs.[10]

One fascinating case study described a psychiatric patient with a split personality. As one personality, the patient was not diabetic and her blood glucose levels were normal. However, the moment she became her alter ego, she *believed* she was diabetic, and she literally *became* diabetic. Her entire physiology shifted. Her blood sugars rose, and from all medical evidence, she was, in fact, diabetic. When her personality flipped back, her blood sugars returned to normal.[11]

Psychiatrist Bennett Braun, author of *The Treatment of Multiple Personality Disorder,* describes several similar cases. Timmy, for example, drinks orange juice uneventfully. But Timmy is only one of one patient's many personalities, and while Timmy can drink orange juice without consequence, all the other personalities are allergic to orange juice and break out into blistering hives at the slightest sip. If, however, Timmy comes back in the midst of an allergic reaction, the hives instantly resolve, and the water-filled blisters begin to subside.[12]

Nocebos can result in sickness, and even death, when the patient expects such an outcome. Scientific studies investigating the nocebo effect can be ethically challenging, since it's hard to get institutional review boards to approve studies designed to intentionally make patients feel worse. Because of this, there is less data to support the existence of the nocebo effect than the placebo effect. Most of what we know about the nocebo effect comes as a side effect of clinical trials that include placebos.

When patients in double-blinded clinical trials are warned about the side effects they may experience if they're given the real drug, approximately 25 percent do experience side effects, sometimes severe, even when they're only taking sugar pills.[13] Those treated with nothing more than placebos often report fatigue, vomiting, muscle weakness, colds, ringing in the ears, taste disturbances, memory disturbances, and other symptoms that shouldn't result from a sugar pill.

Interestingly, these nocebo complaints aren't random; they tend to arise in response to the side-effect warnings on the actual drug or treatment. The mere suggestion that a patient may experience negative symptoms in response to a medication (or a sugar pill) may be a self-fulfilling prophecy. For example, if you tell a patient treated with a placebo he might experience nausea, he's likely to feel nauseous. If you suggest that he might get a headache, he may. In other words, the power of suggestion is *powerful.*[14]

The nocebo effect is probably most obvious in "voodoo death," when a person is cursed and told he or she will die, then dies.[15] The notion of voodoo death doesn't just apply to witch doctors in tribal cultures. The literature shows that patients believed to be terminal who are mistakenly informed that they have only a few months to live have died within their given time frame, even when autopsy findings reveal no physiological explanation for the early death.[16]

Dr. Sanford Cohen described an AIDS patient who experts believe died because he overheard his mother saying she wanted him to die. The patient, whose mother learned on the same day that her son was both gay and afflicted with AIDS, openly prayed outside his ICU room that he would die because of the shame he brought on her. One hour later, he did die, much to the doctor's surprise, since the patient had not appeared to be terminal.[17]

Some believe that those who suffer from premenstrual syndrome (PMS) symptoms may be victims of a sort of nocebo effect. Because they believe they will experience symptoms before their menses, they do. One study of women debilitated by PMS engineered a scheme to trick the study subjects into thinking their periods would come at a different time than they normally expected by giving them an inert pill they were told would alter the timing of their menses. For example, a woman who normally gets her period mid-month and suffers from PMS for three days before her menses was told she would menstruate on the first of the month instead.

What happened? Even though the timing of her period didn't actually change, she got her PMS early that month because she *believed* she would.[18]

Nocebo symptoms can manifest in large groups as well as individuals. For example, after the nuclear power plant disaster in Japan following the 2011 tsunami, people with no evidence of radiation exposure reported symptoms of radiation poisoning as far away as the United States. Similarly, thousands of people with no evidence of disease reported symptoms of swine flu after the media blasted reports of the epidemic all over the television, newspapers, and Internet. Similar "epidemics" have been reported in workplaces, schools, and towns where gas leaks, strange odors, or insect bites have been reported in the media.[19]

So how does this happen? How can someone shed hair when given saline? How can they vomit when given sugar water? How can they become diabetic or allergic to orange juice just by switching personalities? What is occurring, both in the brain and in the body? I kept digging to find my answers.

Scientists believe the nocebo effect is caused primarily by activation of the same stress response the placebo effect relieves. When a patient is cursed, either by a witch doctor, a family member, or a modern physician, the stress of the bad news stimulates the stress response. For example, when patients were told they would experience pain (but were given only an inert substance), the HPA axis was stimulated, increasing cortisol levels. Both pain and excess stimulation of the HPA axis were experienced and then relieved with Valium, indicating that a stress mechanism was at play.[20]

Some also theorize that those who are pronounced ill may become so despondent that they simply stop caring for themselves and suffer the consequences of poor self-care. They may also become depressed, and as I'll discuss in Chapter 7, the link between depression and poor health is very clear.

You Are Not a Victim of Your Genes

Further support for the idea that our beliefs translate into physiological changes in our bodies comes from the laboratories of those studying the field of molecular biology called epigenetics, meaning "control above the genes." So what's "above the genes" when we talk about epigenetic control?

Yup. You guessed it. The mind. As it turns out, while you can't change your DNA, you may be able to utilize the power of your mind to alter how your DNA expresses itself. Traditional genetic determinism, as elucidated by Watson and Crick, who discovered the DNA double helix, supports the notion that everything in the body is controlled by our genes—that essentially, our genes are our destiny. If this is true, we are literally victims of our genes. Heart disease, breast cancer, alcoholism, depression, high cholesterol—you name it. If it runs in your family, you're basically hosed.

The dogma of genetic determinism, as it has been traditionally taught, is simple. You're born with your DNA, which then gets replicated as RNA before being translated into a protein. But the study of epigenetics is uncovering new theories that bring the whole notion of genetic determinism into question.

Scientists now believe that external signals—things like nutrition, the environment in which we live, even thoughts and emotions—can influence regulatory proteins that determine how and even whether DNA gets expressed in certain ways. In other words, it's not as cut and dried as we once thought.

There's more and more science coming out about the physiology of what happens when you believe you will get well versus when you believe you will be sick. Yet, for many of us, our thoughts about our health stem from our childhoods, when negative thoughts about our health may have been programmed into our minds against our will.

Sadly, most of us are not programmed to have positive thoughts about our health. Instead, from the time we are children, our minds get programmed with beliefs that sabotage our efforts to become optimally healthy and happy. Beliefs like "I catch colds easily," "I always overeat," "I probably won't live very long," and "Cancer runs in my family" cause the mind to trigger physiological mechanisms that harm the body.

These programmed beliefs that arise from childhood apply not just to physical health. They also apply to deeper and broader self-limiting beliefs ("I'm not worthy," "I'm not smart enough," "I don't deserve to make a lot of money," "I'm a loser," "Nobody will ever love me").

A Closer Look at Epigenetics

As it turns out, changing your thoughts can actually change how your brain communicates with the rest of your body, thereby altering the body's biochemistry. It's not just your brain that is subject to this kind of plasticity. While you can't change your DNA, cell biologist and author Dr. Bruce Lipton asserts that you may be able to change how your DNA is expressed based on what you believe.[21]

Your genetic code is like a blueprint that can be interpreted in millions of different ways. Before the Human Genome Project, biologists assumed that we had at least 120,000 genes, one gene for every protein made in the body. So researchers were baffled when they discovered that we only have approximately 25,000 genes, which can express themselves in a variety of different ways.

In fact, we now know that each of those 25,000 genes can express itself in at least 30,000 ways via regulatory proteins that are influenced by environmental signals. (Do the math!) Studies have even shown that environmental factors can override certain genetic mutations, effectively changing how the DNA is expressed. These altered genes can then be passed down to offspring, allowing the offspring to express healthier characteristics, even though they still carry the genetic mutation.[22]

The study of epigenetic control is revolutionizing how we think about genes. We used to think that some people were blessed with "good genes," while others were cursed with what some in the medical community insensitively refer to as "piss-poor protoplasm." In fact, few diseases result from a single gene mutation. Less than 2 percent of diseases, such as cystic fibrosis, Huntington's chorea, and beta thalassemia, result from a single faulty gene, and only about 5 percent of cancer and cardiac-disease patients can attribute their diseases to heredity.[23] Scientists are now learning that the genome is far more responsive to the environment of the cell than genetic determinism suggests. This means that the majority of disease processes can be explained by environmental factors to which the cells are exposed, things such as nutrition, hormonal changes, and even love. We need not be victims of our DNA.

The Body as a Petri Dish

Intrigued by what I learned in Lipton's book but curious to know more, I interviewed him. He explained to me that in his bench research as a cell biologist, he worked with pleuripotential stem cells, cells that can become anything when they grow up. He placed one cell in a Petri dish, where it was nourished with cell-culture medium, as it divided into many genetically identical cells. Lipton then split the cells into three Petri dishes and exposed them to three different culture mediums (the environment). What he discovered was that the environment to which the cell was exposed determined whether the cell became a muscle cell or a fat cell or a bone cell. Even though all the cells were genetically identical, they expressed themselves differently. The final outcome of the same genetically identical DNA was expressed as radically different cells.

What controlled the fate of the cells? Not the genetics. They were all genetically identical. The sole difference was the environment to which the same DNA was exposed. The cellular environment also determined whether or not the cells stayed healthy. Cells exposed to a "good" environment (a healthy cell medium) enjoyed optimal health, while those exposed to a "bad" environment (an unhealthy cell medium) got sick.

Lipton said, "If I were an allopathic physician of cells, I'd diagnose the cells in the bad medium as sick. Surely, they need medicine. But that's not really what they need. If you take the sick cells out of the bad environment and put them back into the good environment, they naturally recover—without medicine."

One day, as he was observing the cells in his lab, Lipton had an epiphany. He realized that the human body is no different from the cells in his lab. Lipton said, "The human is nothing more than a skin-covered Petri dish with a community of 50 trillion cells. Whether the cells are in our bodies or in the Petri dish doesn't matter. The culture medium of the cells in our bodies is the blood that bathes and feeds them. If we change the composition of the blood, it's the same as changing the culture medium of the cells. So what controls the composition of the blood? The brain is the chemist changing the environment to which our cells are exposed. The brain releases neuropeptides, hormones, growth factors, and other chemicals, akin to adding chemicals to a Petri dish with a pipette, thereby changing the cell medium."

When I asked him how belief can change the cellular environment, Lipton explained that the brain is perception, but the mind is interpretation. It's all about how the mind interprets a life event. For example, you can open your eyes and see a person. (This is your brain's objective perception.) Your mind may then recognize this person as someone you love. (This is the mind's interpretation.) The brain then releases oxytocin, dopamine, endorphins, and other positive chemicals that provide the healthy cell medium of the whole body's cells via the blood.

If, on the other hand, you open your eyes and see a person (the perception), and your mind interprets this person as scary, the brain releases stress hormones and other fear chemicals that damage the cells. Lipton says, "When we shift the mind's interpretation of illness from fear and danger to positive belief, the brain responds biochemically, the blood changes the body's cell culture, and the cells change on a biological level."

I had my own aha moment when Dr. Lipton explained this to me. Suddenly, it was all making sense. It all kept coming back to the hormones and neurotransmitters the brain spits out, depending on whether the mind interprets something as positive (as it does with the placebo effect) or negative (as with the nocebo effect). When our beliefs are hopeful and optimistic, the mind releases chemicals that put the body in a state of physiological rest, controlled primarily by the parasympathetic nervous system, and in this state of rest, the body's natural self-repair mechanisms are free to get to work fixing what's broken in the body.

If, however, the mind thinks negative beliefs, the brain perceives these as a threat. As far as the brain is concerned, there's a lion running after you, so it's time to fight and flee. When the body's stress responses are activated, the body isn't concerned with long-term issues like cellular rejuvenation, self-repair, and fighting the effects of aging. It's too busy preparing you to run away from the lion. No point putting your immune cells to work chewing up stray cancer cells or turning over fresh new cells in the body if you're about to get eaten.

Over time, these negative beliefs that repetitively trigger the stress response take their toll. The cellular environment gets poisoned with stress hormones. It's no wonder the body gets sick and has a hard time repairing itself.

What Happened in the Womb Matters

Environmental factors can affect how DNA expresses itself as far back as when we were in the womb. A wide range of diseases that affect adults—like osteoporosis and depression—have been linked to prenatal and perinatal developmental influences.[24] Once again, this throws the whole notion of genetic determinism into question.

In *Life in the Womb,* Dr. Peter Nathanielsz explains that there is mounting evidence that programming of lifetime health by the conditions of the womb is as important as, if not more important than, our genes in determining how we perform mentally and physically during life. He calls this limited view of genetics *gene myopia.*[25]

The affection we receive in infancy also shapes our baby brains, changing receptors in the brain, which affect the thermostat of how the adult body responds to stressful stimuli, which in turn can translate into disease in later life. In fact, lack of mother-baby bonding in early life not only affects our bodies; it may threaten our whole society, predisposing it to depression, aggression, and drug abuse, thereby affecting the peace of an entire culture.[26]

In other words, our parents can shape our health when we're barely more than a twinkle in their eyes. A whole host of chronic diseases can develop as the result of adverse environmental influences we experience as fetuses.[27]

Your Subconscious Mind

Our parents also shape the beliefs that reside in our subconscious minds. Negative beliefs we observe in our parents get involuntarily programmed into our subconscious minds at a young age, beliefs like "You're weak" or "You're going to wind up fat and saddled with diabetes when you grow up." Your subconscious mind gets filled with beliefs you download from parents, teachers, and others who influence you early in life, filling your mind with the programs that will run your life unless you learn to reprogram your subconscious mind. Usually, by the age of six, these programs are written, and few people ever make efforts to examine and rewrite their subconscious programming. Given that we have no control over how this powerful part of our brain gets programmed when we're children, it's no wonder most people struggle to change limiting and self-sabotaging beliefs that can harm not just their health, but all aspects of their lives.

Even if the conscious mind of your adult self is filled with positive, hopeful thoughts, you operate from the subconscious mind 95 percent of the time. These habitual negative beliefs, which kick in anytime we're not focusing our attention on positive thoughts, become the default. They operate when we're sleeping, when we're working, or anytime we're not consciously repeating our positive affirmations. Such beliefs may then activate a type of nocebo effect, since if the subconscious mind believes we will get sick, the brain perceives a threat and the stress response is triggered. Next thing you know, your body is busy running away from that perceived lion again, and the body suffers.

The power of the subconscious mind explains why positive thinking only gets you so far. How many times have you read self-help books, taken workshops, made New Year's resolutions, and vowed to improve your life, only to realize a year later that your life is no better? Since the conscious mind is only functioning 5 percent of the time, it has little power to overcome the weighty influence of the subconscious mind. To effect lasting changes in belief, you must change your beliefs not just at the level of the conscious mind, but in the subconscious mind.

Be Mindful of How You Program Children

Many of us were programmed to have disempowering thoughts about our health at an early age. Few of our parents taught us that our minds have the power to heal and harm our own bodies. Instead, we were programmed to believe that our bodies are none of our business, that we have little to no power to help ourselves get well.

As children, most of us learn that when the body gets sick, we must go to the doctor and get treated. When a child falls and skins her knee, rarely does the parent say, "Okay honey. Now your knee can focus on healing itself." No! We race off to get ointments and Band-Aids. There's nothing wrong with ointments and Band-Aids, but they feed into the child's erroneous belief that the body is dependent on treatments that come from the outside, rather than the self-repair mechanisms our bodies all have naturally. As adults, we wind up believing we are powerless to control the outcomes of our health, when really we are infinitely powerful.

I was a victim of such programming myself. As a child, salty foods, rather than sweets, were my biggest weaknesses. I loved soup, chips, cheese, anything savory, and my mother always told me that if I ate a lot of salt, I was going to have high blood pressure when I grew up. Nobody in my family has high blood pressure. Mom and Dad both had unusually low blood pressure, in fact. But my subconscious mind was programmed to believe I would grow up and have high blood pressure.

So it was no surprise to me when, as a skinny, 20-something, otherwise healthy woman with no family history of high blood pressure, I was diagnosed with hypertension.

It wasn't until years later, when I started studying the power of positive and negative belief, that I realized what my own subconscious beliefs might have created. Could it be coincidence? Was I destined to get high blood pressure anyway? Maybe. Nobody can say for sure. But it makes you wonder . . .

Imagine if parents programmed impressionable young subconscious minds to believe we have self-healing superpowers to fight disease and activate health, instead of teaching us that illness must be treated by dosing us up with medication every time we get sick and hauling us off to the doctor's office for a shot. Imagine how optimally healthy our subconscious minds would be.

What I've learned has changed how I parent my daughter, Siena. When she was three or four, before I learned what I now know, my husband, Matt, would joke with Siena when she got sick or injured. Mimicking an ambulance siren, he would race around the room with her in his arms, yelling, "Quick! Somebody call the ambulance! We have to take Siena to the kid factory so we can get her a new leg" (or lip or nose). She would laugh, and we would cover her injury with a Band-Aid or take her to the doctor. But the underlying message we were programming into her subconscious mind was "You have to go to the kid factory in order to get better." With that kind of programming, it would be hard for her adult self to accept that the body can heal itself.

Until I started researching the self-healing process, Matt and I had no idea we might be inadvertently affecting Siena's health and well-being. Certainly, my mother never wanted anything for her children but health and happiness. Most of us just don't realize how we're programming our children and the consequences this may have in later life.

Now, Matt and I have altered how we speak about illness, injury, and the healing process to Siena. If she wakes up with a tummy ache, we remind her that she has the power to heal herself and then often treat her with a placebo—a cough drop or a Tic Tac—or sometimes a dose of cold medicine or a homeopathic remedy. When we give her the pill, we remind her, "This is just to help you heal yourself."

After we started doing this, she began speaking of illness and injury in a whole new way. She'd fall down and skin her knee, but then she'd jump right up and say, "Don't worry, Mommy. My knee knows how to heal itself."

My husband and I have certainly never withheld medical treatment from our child when she needs it—and that's not what I'm suggesting at all. If, God forbid, Siena were ever diagnosed with a serious illness, we'd be racing off to the doctor's office lickety-split. But we've found that Siena almost never needs to visit the doctor for anything other than routine checkups. Plus, she now bounces back much more quickly from the cold and flu viruses she brings home from kindergarten. Perhaps, when she's older, our childhood programming of her subconscious mind will make it easier for her to overcome any resistance of her mind to the process of self-healing.

But what about you? What if your parents never programmed your subconscious mind to believe it could heal itself? What if you want to believe your mind can heal your body, but you just don't? If you feel hopeless or discouraged, don't despair. The good news is that negative beliefs about health, which trigger nocebo effects and lead to poor health, can be reprogrammed. (For more about how to change subconscious beliefs from negative ones to positive ones, see Chapter 10.)

Medical Hexing

Once we change our beliefs on a subconscious level, we optimize the culture medium for the community of cells that make up the human body, thereby changing the way our DNA expresses itself. We are not victims of our genes. We are masters of our own destiny.

The data proving this was so compelling, yet part of me began to feel irresponsible for not knowing about this sooner. When I recited the Hippocratic Oath, I promised to "First, do no harm." I started feeling guilty for any role I might have played in inadvertently harming my patients, both by failing to educate them about how their beliefs could manifest physically and by projecting my own beliefs onto them and possibly hurting them unwittingly.

When we pronounce upon someone with statistics like "Nine out of ten people with your condition die in six months" or "You have a twenty percent chance of five-year survival," is this far from the voodoo practices of some native cultures? Are we cursing them, triggering fear responses in their mind, and causing their minds to activate stress responses, when the body most needs relaxation responses?

When we pronounce our patients "incurable" or even label them with a "chronic" disease like multiple sclerosis or Crohn's disease or high blood pressure, and we tell them they will be afflicted their whole lives, are we not, in essence, harming them? What proof do we have that they will not be one of the case studies who winds up in the Spontaneous Remission Project, having been cured of a so-called incurable illness?

In *Spontaneous Healing,* Dr. Andrew Weil argues that physicians may unwittingly engage in what he calls "medical hexing." When we pronounce that patients have "chronic," "incurable," or "terminal" illnesses, we may be programming their subconscious minds with negative beliefs and activating stress responses that do more harm than good. By labeling a patient with a negative prognosis and robbing him or her of the hope that cure might be possible, we may ultimately prove the poor prognosis we have bestowed upon our patient correct. Wouldn't we be better off offering hope and triggering the mind to release health-inducing chemicals intended to aid the body's self-repair mechanisms?

When my father was diagnosed with metastatic melanoma, complete with brain and liver metastases, the news was grim. As doctors, Dad and I both knew the stats—less than 5 percent of people with Dad's condition survived five years, and most died within three to six months.

Looking back and knowing what I now know, I honestly wish we hadn't known those numbers when we found out Dad had melanoma in his brain. With one look at the numbers, hope was dashed—for both of us. We never focused on the 5 percent of people who actually survive. And who's to say Dad couldn't have been one of them? All we could think about was the 95 percent who died—usually very quickly.

Now, after all I've learned, I realize that doctors who deliver these kinds of numbers to patients may in fact be inadvertently harming their patients. We can't see the future. We have no way to predict which patients will defy the odds and which will succumb quickly. Our intentions are pure. We are motivated by honesty, a commitment to patient autonomy, and the desire to prepare our patients for the worst so they don't wander around in a state of denial.

But if the patient is the one out of ten who doesn't die, have we done him or her any favors by warning of something that might never come to pass? Is our desire for full disclosure worth eliminating hope and shattering beliefs, just so our patients can be "realistic" about their prognosis?

I'm not suggesting that we return to the old-school paternalistic model of "Don't worry your pretty little head over it, ma'am." In early 20th-century medicine, doctors would hide a patient's medical condition from the patient because "If Grandma knew, it would just kill her."

Nope. Honesty and collaboration are cornerstones of the doctor-patient relationship and mustn't be tampered with. Education, empowerment, and full disclosure are definitely my modus operandi. But I do question how we deliver the information. Doesn't it make sense for all of us—healers and patients alike—to shift how we think and communicate so we can optimize the body's chance for optimal health?

As a physician, here's what I've learned: somewhere in the intersection of hope, optimism, nurturing care, and full partnership with the empowered patient, a recipe for healing lies.

Chapter 3

THE HEALING FACTOR THAT CAN MAKE ALL THE DIFFERENCE

"The secret of the care of the patient is in caring for the patient."

— FRANCIS PEABODY

I remember one day when Mom called me, complaining of severe pain in her abdomen. She had been suffering from bloating and bouts of diarrhea since Dad died, but this pain in her belly was new. Mom sounded scared. I reassured her as much as I could from 3,000 miles away.

I scrolled through the differential diagnosis in my mind. Was it her gallbladder? A bleeding ulcer? Pancreatitis? A strange presentation of appendicitis? A bowel obstruction? A hiatal hernia? Reflux?

I peppered her with the requisite questions. Did she have a fever? Had she vomited? When did she last move her bowels? Was she passing gas? Did she feel hungry?

Her answers led me to believe it was not a surgical emergency. I told her so, but still recommended that she call her primary-care doctor. A few minutes later, Mom called me back. She had paged her doctor, and her doctor had asked her to meet her at the office right away.

It was a long drive to the doctor's office—almost an hour. Halfway through the drive, Mom called me and I asked how she was feeling. The pain had eased a bit. Fifteen minutes later, she had almost arrived at the doctor's office when she called me and said, "Would you believe this darn pain is almost gone?"

By the time she arrived, the pain had disappeared completely.

Mom called me and said, "I swear, this happens to me *all the time*. I want the symptoms to be severe when I get to the doctor's office so they can see me at my worst and help me figure out what's wrong, but more often than not, my symptoms go away before they even call my name."

Bingo.

My mother's doctor never did figure out why she was having the pain, but my conversation with her led me to develop a theory. My mother trusts doctors. She believes they have the power to make her well. Many times, she has felt poorly, and after seeing doctors, she has felt better. Her mind is now firmly convinced that doctors will help her. And because she chooses her health-care providers carefully, Mom genuinely loves her physicians and feels loved by them in return.

But what if the physical improvement she experiences when she goes to the doctor is primarily the result of her mind and its effect on her body? When Mom calls the doctor and makes an appointment, what if her mind registers relaxation, hope, optimism, tenderness, and the belief that healing is on the way? Her brain lets out a huge sigh of relief. Her thoughts shut down the stress responses she experienced when she first noticed the pain, the idea of visiting the doctor elicits a relaxation response, the body rests, and her natural self-repair mechanisms get activated. Before she knows it, the body has taken care of the problem, and voilà! The symptoms are gone.

The trip to the doctor winds up getting all the credit, but the real hero is her own mind.

Of course, this not to diminish what doctors can do. When my husband cut two fingers off his hand with a table saw, and his doctor, Dr. Jonathan Jones, stitched them back on with advanced microsurgical techniques, Matt and I were in full-on worship mode. This brilliant man, who came in on his day off, used a microscope to sew back together every artery, nerve, and bone in Matt's fingers so my husband, an artist and a writer, could still use his hands. I was so grateful to my physician colleague that I made him a painting of my own hand, as a gesture of my respect for the skill, love, commitment, and devotion he had shown to my husband.

But as much as I'm grateful to Dr. Jones, I credit Matt with much of his recovery. From the get-go, Matt held a belief that his fingers would be sewed back on and work as well as they did before he lost them. He had perfect faith in modern medicine, and even after cutting his fingers off, he looked at me with wide eyes and said, "It's all going to be okay." He felt no pain during the incident, probably because his body was full of pain-relieving endorphins, and when I called 911 and the paramedics arrived, Matt expressed relief. I can only imagine that his brain was spitting out healing hormones and health-inducing chemicals that aided his recovery and made Dr. Jones's job easier, but the truth of the matter is that someone still had to sew those fingers back on. They weren't going to replant themselves.

When doctors save us, especially when we are facing life- or limb-threatening traumas or diseases, it's tempting to lift them up on pedestals and give them all the credit. And yes, some doctors are exceptionally gifted, and what they do speeds up the healing process so the body can go about the business of self-repair. But when the surgeon cuts out a tumor or prescribes an antibiotic or sets a broken bone, we still depend on the body's self-repair mechanisms to finish the job. Matt's body still had to fuse those reconnected bones and heal those cuts in his arteries and nerves. Dr. Jones made it possible for his body to do so.

I want to make it clear that, when I talk about the body's ability to repair itself, I am in no way suggesting that we should forego the advances modern medicine now makes available to us. While I believe our bodies have a remarkable capacity for self-repair, I also believe we shouldn't expect our bodies to do all the heavy lifting, and sometimes, the body will simply fail if we expect it to do all the work.

While my mother might not have needed her doctor's touch to cure her belly pain, Matt clearly needed Dr. Jones. Sometimes we rely on the technology modern medicine has to offer, and sometimes we don't. But I can promise you this: in either scenario, finding the right person to support your healing journey is crucial, and the scientific data I studied confirms this.

The Doctor as Medicine

Patients get well, at least in part, because they believe in the power of modern medicine and expect to feel relief when they see doctors and other health-care specialists they trust. My mother and Matt are not alone in placing great faith and trust in doctors. Many people experience similar conditioned responses when visiting the doctor. Patients become accustomed to going to the doctor and subsequently feeling better, so the mind may work its magic before the therapeutic encounter has actually happened, even with no direct therapeutic intervention.

But what does the scientific data show?

I went back to the medical journals, and from what I learned, a nurturing therapeutic relationship may be responsible for a large part of the positive response patients experience when treated with placebos. Scientists postulate that it wouldn't be enough to just imbibe placebos if they were self-administered without the participation of a physician—that to be truly powerful, someone in whom the patient places great faith must deliver them.

In an interview on NPR, Ted Kaptchuk, director of Harvard's Program in Placebo Studies and the Therapeutic Encounter (PiPS), said, "A sugar pill doesn't do anything. What does something is the context of healing. It's the rituals of healing. It's being in a healing relationship . . . But the placebo pill is a wonderful tool, or a saline injection is a wonderful tool, to isolate what is usually in the background, take it away from the medications and procedures that medicine does, and actually study just the act of caring. That's, I think, what we're measuring when we study placebo effects."[1]

When Kaptchuk, who is trained as a Chinese medicine practitioner and acupuncturist, was asked how he, as a scientist, justified practicing acupuncture when most randomized, controlled clinical trials failed to demonstrate its effectiveness beyond placebo, he said, "Because I am a damn good healer. That is the difficult truth. If you needed help and you came to me, you would get better. Thousands of people have. Because, in the end, it isn't really about the needles. It's about the man."[2]

Kaptchuk's sentiments are affirmed in the *New England Journal of Medicine* article he co-wrote, which studied asthmatics. Those who reported being short of breath were treated with an albuterol inhaler (standard treatment for asthma), a sham inhaler (placebo), fake acupuncture (also placebo), and no treatment. All of the treated patients felt equally better—approximately 50 percent improvement for those treated with albuterol, the sham inhaler, and the fake acupuncture, compared to a 21 percent improvement in those receiving no treatment.

However, unlike other studies, which demonstrated physiological responses that coincided with symptomatic relief, when researchers in this study measured lung function in the asthmatics, the physiological response did not equal the patient's subjective experience. The lung function measured in those who received fake acupuncture, a sham inhaler, and no treatment all experienced improved lung function (7 percent) but not nearly as much as those getting albuterol (20 percent).[3]

Why were these asthmatics feeling better, even when their bodies weren't demonstrating physiological responses to explain the clinical improvement? Perhaps patients in the study were feeling better, not just because of the albuterol, fake acupuncture, or sham inhaler, but because *somebody cared.* What if the patients were treated not by the medicine itself, but by the medical care? Perhaps the treatment groups felt equally better because they received equal care, and perhaps that's even more important than the drug or treatment they receive.

Asthma may be different from cancer. When you're battling a life-threatening illness, it's not so much the symptom relief you're after; it's the disease remission. Is the cancer gone or not? But what if symptom relief and disease remission are linked by the therapeutic experience and its relationship to the mind, the damages of the stress response, and the healing power of the relaxation response?

I suspected there was a potent link, but once again, I wanted proof.

Proof That Nurturing Care Makes a Difference

At this point in my research, I strongly suspected that a huge part of the placebo effect revolved around the delivery of nurturing care. And I had a sneaking suspicion that lack of loving care—especially with regard to medical hexing—could elicit nocebo effects. But how much of an effect did it have, and was there any evidence that the bedside manner or beliefs of the health-care provider affected health outcomes?

Dr. Lawrence Egbert conducted a study at Harvard Medical School, published in the *New England Journal of Medicine,* for which he randomized preoperative surgical patients into two groups. One group met with cheerful, optimistic anesthesiologists who assured them that their surgery was going to be a piece of cake, they were going to be comfortable and pain-free, and everything was going to be peachy. The other unfortunate patients (poor babies!) were attended by anesthesiologists instructed to be grumpy, rushed, and unsympathetic. (Interestingly, they were actually the same anesthesiologists wearing two different hats.) Those who got the optimistic anesthesiologists required only half the amount of painkilling medication and were discharged an average of 2.6 days earlier.[4]

Optimism on the part of the physician also makes a difference. Fueled by the comment, "The reason why Dr. Smith is so successful is because he's so positive," in 1987, Dr. K. B. Thomas was inspired to conduct a study on whether a physician's positive attitude affects patient outcomes. His study, conducted at the University of Southampton and published in the *British Medical Journal* evaluated 200 of his own patients who didn't feel well but didn't have any apparent abnormalities on examination. The patients were randomly selected to receive one of four different types of consultations: a consultation conducted in a "positive manner," with and without treatment, and a consultation conducted in a "non-positive manner," with and without treatment. Sixty-four percent of those receiving a positive consultation got better, compared with 39 percent of those who received a negative consultation. The study found that patient recovery could be increased by words that suggested the patient "would be better in a few days" and, if he were given treatment, that "the treatment would certainly make him better." On the flip side, negative words such as "I am not sure that the treatment I am going to give you will have an effect" led to longer recovery times.[5] Thomas concluded, "The doctor himself is a powerful therapeutic agent; he is the placebo and his influence is felt to a greater or lesser extent at every consultation."[6]

While optimism and positive words are key, trust is just as important. Nocebo effects can occur when a patient distrusts medical personnel and the therapies they implement.[7] I used to work in a public health clinic in San Diego, where most of my patients were Somali refugees. Coming from a culture where medicine is practiced much differently, many of my patients were deeply distrusting of American doctors and the treatments we prescribed. In this patient population, I witnessed far more side effects resulting from common, seemingly innocuous treatments, such as prenatal vitamins, than my American patients usually reported. Although I worked hard to earn the trust of these patients, I suspect these side effects occurred because some of them genuinely believed we were trying to poison them.

What your doctor believes also matters. In a study published in the *Lancet,* which investigated the role of endorphins in how placebos relieve pain, researchers found that, despite the use of a double-blind procedure, the expectations of the physicians still influenced how patients responded to injections of fentanyl, naloxone, or placebo.[8] If the doctor doesn't believe a certain treatment will work, the treatment may actually be less effective.

Another study conducted by the National Institute of Mental Health assessed 250 depressed patients who were randomized to one of four 16-week treatment groups: interpersonal psychotherapy, cognitive behavior therapy, the antidepressant imipramine, and placebo. As a sub-study of the larger project, researchers at Georgetown videotaped how doctors participating in this study interacted with patients and, based on these video exchanges, asked expert raters to predict who would get well and who wouldn't.

Surprisingly, these raters were able to predict this, based on the doctor-patient relationship, regardless of which treatment the patient was given. It wasn't just whether or not the doctor and patient connected emotionally. It turns out that what the doctor believed about the patient's prognosis also turned out to be crucial. If a doctor believed that the patient would improve, he or she was more likely to do so than if the doctor did not radiate this type of positivity.[9] These findings about physician beliefs have since been replicated in many other studies, not just in the field of mental health, but in other areas.

Not surprisingly, the personality of the physician makes a difference as well. A Harvard Medical School study published in the *British Medical Journal* demonstrated that the response to a placebo increased from 44 percent to 62 percent when the doctor treated the patient with "warmth, attention, and confidence." Among a third control group of people on a waiting list who received no medical care at all, only 28 percent improved.[10]

The right support, combined with positive belief, can even result in inexplicable cure. In the early 1950s, Dr. Albert Mason at the Queen Victoria Hospital in London treated a teenage boy with thick, cracked leathery skin covering most of his body. His condition was believed to be a severe case of warts, and since hypnosis had previously been described as an effective treatment for warts, Dr. Mason genuinely believed hypnosis could cure the warts, even at such an advanced stage.[11]

Convinced of the mind's power to induce self-repair of warts, Dr. Mason got to work. During the first session, Dr. Mason focused solely on the boy's arm, bringing the boy into a trance state and guiding him through the process of seeing his arm as pink and healthy. After repeated treatment, the skin was nearly normal, to the shock and awe of Dr. Mason's peers. But Dr. Mason wasn't surprised. He had faith that the mind could heal the body, at least for a condition like severe warts.

When the boy was then seen by his surgeon, who had unsuccessfully tried to help the boy with skin grafts, the surgeon was amazed to see the boy's healthy skin, especially because the surgeon had made a mistake. Instead of suffering from warts, the boy had been misdiagnosed. His real condition was a severe, potentially lethal genetic condition called congenital ichthyosis.

Although no evidence had ever demonstrated that the mind could cure congenital ichthyosis, both Dr. Mason and the boy believed hypnosis would work. And it did.

Word got out and others who suffered from congenital ichthyosis sought out Dr. Mason, who tried to help them. But Dr. Mason was unable to later replicate the same effect in others. He blamed his failure on his own lack of belief. While he believed hypnosis would cure warts, he doubted its efficacy for this more serious genetic condition, even though hypnosis had already cured it once.

The Ritual of Medicine

A sugar pill, while powerful, is really just a sugar pill. It's not magic. While some treatments, like my husband's hand surgery, repair the body in ways the body could not induce alone, other treatments merely enlist the mind's potent power to optimize the health of the body, and the support of a caring health-care provider makes all the difference.

Some studies—like K. B. Thomas's—go so far as to suggest that the doctor is, in fact, the placebo, that the role the physician plays, in and of itself, triggers the self-healing response.[12] What we've learned from the placebo effect is that, as Ted Kaptchuk explains, the placebo strips away the actual treatments we assume cure us—the antibiotics, the knee surgery, the antidepressants, the painkillers, the chest surgery—distilling medicine down to something therapeutic that has less to do with pills or surgery. Without the biochemical trappings of medicine, we're left only with medicine as it used to be back before highly effective treatments like Matt's finger surgery existed—the ritual of medicine, the meaning we ascribe to the medical treatment, and the care of someone devoted to trying to help us get well.

Because the role of the physician in the Western world has been imbued with so much meaning in our modern culture, the support of a caring physician may carry even more weight than the same kind of support from a pastor, therapist, acupuncturist, or other loving, healing presence. Yet the same might not be true in other cultures, where the greatest healing power may lie with the shaman, the Chinese medicine doctor, or the medicine woman.

One doctor I interviewed—we'll call her Dr. M—said, "I know that the most valuable thing I offer my patients is love." She told me a story about a patient with severe nerve pain that plagued 90 percent of her body. The patient had seen dozens of physicians and quite a few alternative medicine healers, without relief. Then she saw Dr. M, who prescribed fish oil and B vitamins. Dr. M admitted to me that she prescribed the supplements mostly as a placebo, because there was no clinical evidence to support the idea that they would be effective against this nerve pain. She also spent hours listening to this patient and offering her nurturing care.

Soon afterward, the patient fell head over heels in love with a young man, and shortly thereafter, she returned to Dr. M's office to announce that her pain was gone. She credited the B vitamins and fish oil, calling them a miracle cure.

But Dr. M told me, "I knew it wasn't the vitamins. I believe it was the love of this young man—in combination with the care I offered—that cured her."

The Mechanism of Nurturing Care

How can the nurturing care and positive belief of a health-care provider result in better health of the patient? It all goes back to the illness-inducing stress response and the self-repair-facilitating relaxation response. When a patient who imbues the physician with positive meaning feels tended, trusting, reassured, and nurtured, the stress response is aborted. The relaxation response is induced. The patient starts to get better right away.

Just imagine you're diagnosed with cancer. The minute you hear the word *cancer*, your fight-or-flight stress responses go crazy. The adrenal gland pumps out cortisol. The sympathetic nervous system jumps to attention. The word *cancer* is interpreted by the mind as a deadly threat, even though the threat of death isn't usually imminent at the time of diagnosis. In such a state of physiological stress, the body is poorly equipped to fight cancer. It's too busy preparing to fight and flee.

Then in walks the oncologist, who is kind, nurturing, and reassuring. He holds your hand, hugs you when you cry, and assures you that he has cared for thousands of people with just such a cancer and most of them have done well. With calm words and gentle presence, the oncologist explains that no matter what happens, you will never be alone, that he will be right there by your side, doing everything in his power to help. A treatment plan is made, and he gives you a phone number you can call if you think of any more questions. He offers you another hug or gentle pat on the back. Even though you're facing a big surgery and months of chemotherapy, you feel better already.

Why? Because the mind is soothed. The fear is alleviated. The stress response is turned off. The body relaxes. The doctor convinced your brain that all will be well, or at least that everything will be done to try to ensure that it will be. In such a relaxed state, the body can get busy doing what it does best—making efforts to heal itself.

The Absence of Nurturing Care Can Harm You

So if calming, reassuring doctors who believe all will be well can induce such positive physiological effects, we know what happens when physicians unwittingly use their superpowers in the wrong way. Although they may mean well, all too often, doctors and other health-care providers not only fail to treat their patients with nurturing care and tenderness; they may even allow themselves to get so busy, overworked, and depleted that they flat-out harm their patients.

A friend wrote to me after leaving her doctor's office:

> *Lissa, if this doctor robs me as I leave the building, I won't be able to confirm it was him, as I don't think he looked at me once. From the nurse intake to the actual exam room, both practitioners faced AWAY from me, toward their computer terminals, while they asked me questions and clicked away at the keyboard. The computer fed him my new prescription, and he never even discussed it with me. If a computer program is all I need to monitor and refill prescriptions on my current or chronic conditions, then what am I doing spending an hour in a waiting room, waiting to look at some guy's back? Oh, and don't forget—the nurse clearly put a wrong code into the computer, because he came in prepared to give me a BREAST exam, rather than listening*

to my asthmatic CHEST. I was like, "What are you talking about, sir? You have the wrong information or else the wrong room." Sigh. I'm so mad right now. I'm never coming here ever again.

I've heard this kind of feedback frequently from my online community. With many health-care providers feeling overburdened, exhausted, and unappreciated, patients sometimes wind up feeling more stressed after a doctor's visit than they did before. If you have to sit for two hours in a crowded waiting room, only to have seven and a half minutes with an exhausted doctor who cuts you off, forgets your name, never lays a hand on you, and then scares you with a disconcerting prognosis, you can be sure your stress responses will be activated.

Nobody intends for this to happen. Health-care providers have often sacrificed so much for their patients that they stop being mindful about why they're doing what they were called to do. They think the sacrifices demonstrate the care they have for their patients. But sacrifices are not enough. It's time to put the *care* back in health care. Doctors and other health-care providers need to remember why we do what we do so we can maximize the healing effect we have on our patients. Especially when things go wrong.

How to Deliver Bad News

In 1974, Dr. Clifton Meador told his patient Sam Londe, who suffered from cancer of the esophagus, that his condition was considered fatal. After Dr. Meador broke the news about his death sentence, Sam died quickly, only weeks after his diagnosis.

But an autopsy performed after his death surprised doctors. Very little cancer was found—certainly not enough to kill him. Dr. Meador told the Discovery Health Channel, "He died with cancer, but not from cancer." Why did he die? Perhaps the bad news triggered so much fear that stress responses wreaked havoc in his body. He died because he was told he would die and he *believed* he would die. His negative thoughts translated into real physiological changes.

Decades later, Sam Londe's death still haunts Dr. Meador, who said, "I thought he had cancer. He thought he had cancer. Everybody around him thought he had cancer . . . did I remove hope in some way?"[13]

I suspect that this kind of thing is not uncommon. Of course, doctors never mean to harm patients. Most are motivated by the purest intentions, and we want nothing more than to help our patients heal. But I've heard good doctors give the bad news spiel time and time again. It often goes something like this:

DOOR #1

I'm afraid your cancer is inoperable and is not limited to the one organ we thought it was. In fact, it's in your stomach, your colon, your lymph nodes, and dotted all over the lining of your abdomen. We haven't done the studies yet, but it may also be in your lungs, your bones, and your brain.

If you'd like, we can give you chemotherapy, but it will just be palliative, not curative. I'm very sorry to give you this news, and of course, we'll do everything we can to keep you comfortable. But this would be a good time to get your affairs in order. If you haven't updated your will, you might want to do that, because only 1 in 20 people with your kind of cancer survive five years and most die within three to six months.

I'm terribly sorry to have to tell you this, and of course, we can talk further when the effects of the anesthesia have worn off and you're a little more awake.

When bad news is delivered this way, it only triggers stress responses that make it harder for the patient's body to repair itself and, in rare cases, may even lead to death when there is no apparent cause. It's possible that you really can be scared to death.

I propose a new way to deliver bad news. Let's take the same patient we described behind Door #1—the one with metastatic cancer and a 1-in-20 chance of survival. Let's give her some time to wake up from her anesthesia. Let's comfort her in the recovery room. Let's tell the family we'll have a family conference when she fully wakes up, and then let's have this conversation instead:

DOOR #2

I have good news and bad news, so I'll get the bad news out of the way first. I'm afraid the cancer isn't limited to one organ, the way we hoped it would be. [Pause for a moment to give this time to sink in.]

The cancer also appears to have spread to your stomach, your colon, your lymph nodes, and the lining of your abdomen. We'll have to do some tests to see if the cancer might have spread anywhere else, and we should be able to get that information very soon, so we can make a plan about what's next. But I want you to know you will not go through this alone. [Pause again.]

I know that's a lot to hear right now, but let me share with you the good news. The good news is that a percentage of people with exactly this diagnosis survive, and there are some predictors of who those people might be. The body is designed to repair itself when it gets sick, and we have clear evidence that those who nurture their bodies, minds, and spirits while staying hopeful and believing in their ability to get well are more likely to be cured. It's important to your body that we all remain optimistic and that your mind and body stay as relaxed as possible, because only in this state of relaxation can your body fight off the cancer.

I want you to know that I believe that it's possible for you to be cured from this cancer, and I will be here to support you every step of the way. We'll talk tomorrow about treatment options and where we can go from here, but why don't you get some rest first and spend some time processing this with your family. Before I go to do my next surgery, do you have any questions for me right now? [Pause and listen.]

I'll talk to you again first thing in the morning, and if you have any urgent questions that come up between now and then, feel free to give me a call. Here's my number in case you need me. I know this isn't the news you wanted to hear today, but please, never give up hope. I believe in miracles, and you just might be that miracle.

Imagine how differently you would feel after each conversation. The first doctor would likely leave you feeling stressed, uncertain, and upset. The doctor behind Door #2, however, would probably make you feel supported, hopeful, and well informed, so much so that your mind and body are relaxed.

As health-care providers, I think it's our responsibility to consider how we might facilitate the process of helping our patients hold positive beliefs and release negative ones, so we can limit stress responses and elicit relaxation responses that help the body heal itself and prevent further damage. Perhaps this act of love and service will have more profound effects than any drug or surgery. It may take a few more minutes out of our day to deliver bad news in a way that facilitates healing, but the results could be extraordinary.

Physician, Heal Thyself

When health-care professionals hold space with nurturing care, we create the ideal environment for patients to heal themselves. But all too often, we make the mistake of trying to serve those in need of healing from a place of depletion. As doctors, we are taught to sacrifice our own needs in order to serve others. We wind up severely sleep-deprived, we eat poorly, we fail to tend to our relationships, we neglect our self-care, we close our hearts to protect ourselves, and we often wind up physically, emotionally, and spiritually unhealthy. The minute a doctor or other health-care provider gives to the point of depletion, the well is dry, and true healing can no longer happen. Because we are so depleted, we feel victimized, and we wind up becoming the villains, lashing out at patients because we are running on empty.

If I could wave a magic wand and change one thing about the health-care system, I would change the insane notion that, in order to be good health-care providers, we must give at the expense of our own health. It's impossible to be fully present for our patients, to open our hearts as widely as they must be opened, and to serve as fully as we can when we have nothing left to give. If only doctors could be models of self-care so that patients might learn by example, the whole system would undergo a radical shift. If healers could heal themselves first, we would be able to serve and love from a place of wholeness, so we could more effectively heal the world.

15 WAYS HEALERS CAN AMPLIFY THEIR ART

1. Listen.

2. Open your heart.

3. Make eye contact.

4. Take your hand off the doorknob and sit down.

5. Be present.

6. Offer healing touch.

7. Invite your patient to be your partner.

8. Avoid judgment.

9. Educate, but don't dictate.

10. Choose your words with care and remain optimistic.

11. Trust your patient's intuition.

12. Be respectful of other practitioners who are treating your patient.

13. Reassure your patients they are not alone.

14. Encourage stress relief and let your presence relieve stress.

15. Offer hope, because no matter how grim the prognosis, spontaneous remission is always possible.

Healing yourself is hard work, and nobody should have to do it alone. As physicians, we can dose up life-saving treatment, but if we fail to heal ourselves so that we are full enough to sprinkle our treatments with a heaping helping of love, we limit the ability of our patients to fully and sustainably recover.

Norman Cousins, author of *Anatomy of an Illness,* knows this well. Cousins had been diagnosed with the degenerative collagen disorder ankylosing spondylitis, and he believed he would be able to arrest his condition if he were discharged from the hospital and treated with high doses of vitamin C and daily laughter instead of anti-inflammatory drugs, painkillers, and tranquilizers. Fortunately, his doctor, with whom Cousins enjoyed a collaborative partnership based on mutual respect, supported his decision.

In *Anatomy of an Illness,* Cousins wrote, "I would say that the principal contribution made by my doctor to the taming, and possibly the conquest, of my illness was that he encouraged me to believe I was a respected partner with him in the total undertaking."

The Placebo Effect in Complementary and Alternative Medicine

Nurturing care explains why many patients often experience remarkable results when treated by complementary and alternative medicine (CAM) treatments, which include such therapies as acupuncture, Chinese medicine, homeopathy, Reiki, herbal medicine, energy medicine, craniosacral therapy, chiropractic medicine, and other such modalities. Yet CAM treatments are often shown to be "ineffective" according to evidence-based medicine principles—in other words, they're considered no more effective than placebos. I believe the reason many of these treatments have not stood up to placebo-controlled trials is because sham acupuncture, delivered with nurturing care, is as effective as real acupuncture, delivered with nurturing care. Both work equally because, as Kaptchuk stated earlier, it isn't "about the needles." Both trigger relaxation and reduce stress in the body. And this is a good thing, not something CAM healers need to get defensive about!

What if much of what we offer in Western medicine works in the same way? In many cases, especially when it comes to the treatment of "chronic" disease, the care and reassurance we offer is perhaps as valuable to the physiology of the body as the pills and injections.

Please understand, I'm not here to argue whether CAM methods of healing are "effective" or not. If your illness mysteriously vaporized after you took a homeopathic remedy, or if you're an energy healer who has witnessed spontaneous remissions happening to your patients, I do not doubt the efficacy of such treatments. In fact, I fully believe that unexplainable things happen in the hands of trained professionals practicing forms of medicine that scientific data has yet to verify.

Instead of dismissing such treatments, I'd like to make the argument that perhaps nontraditional healing modalities work not so much because of the modality being practiced as because of the potent combination of positive belief in the healing method, the nurturing care offered by the practitioner, and the relaxation responses these treatments induce. Perhaps these modalities are, in fact, highly effective—but not via the means we might expect.

What I'm suggesting is that all interventions aimed at facilitating health and healing—whether conventional drugs and surgeries or CAM treatments—may work primarily through the power of the mind. We've already demonstrated that many conventional medical treatments fare no better than placebo, while others have been proven to be *more* effective than placebo. This suggests that some conventional treatments really do offer benefit beyond what positive belief and nurturing care can facilitate. Most CAM treatments, however, seem to offer most, if not all, of their benefit because of positive belief, nurturing care, and the positive physiological responses they trigger.

Is It the Treatment or the Relaxation Response?

The evidence suggests that real acupuncture may be no more effective than sham acupuncture. A few acupuncture trials demonstrate efficacy beyond sham acupuncture,[14] but the majority do not. When patients were randomized to receive either real acupuncture (inserting needles along energetic meridians as taught in acupuncture school) versus sham acupuncture (inserting needles willy-nilly or poking the skin with fake needles but not sticking them all the way in), many of the people getting real acupuncture got better. But so did the people getting sham acupuncture.[15] Although many people believe it's all about the appropriate needle placement, what if it has more to do with the acupuncturist than the acupuncture technique?

The same is likely true for Reiki, a Japanese form of energy healing typified by laying on hands or waving the hands over the body to move life-force energy through "stuck" places in the body. Studies such as the one conducted at Sonoma State University and published in _Oncology Nursing Forum_ examined patients getting chemotherapy and found that those getting Reiki were more likely to experience positive health outcomes than those getting standard treatment alone, but those getting sham Reiki were equally likely to experience a benefit.[16] Again, this doesn't surprise me. As someone who has practiced Reiki myself, I can attest to the fact that Reiki is profoundly relaxing, especially when it's delivered by someone who really cares. But sham Reiki would be too. No wonder people enjoy it!

Studies also suggest that homeopathy, a CAM therapy based on the hypothesis that a substance that causes the symptoms of a disease in healthy people will cure that disease in sick people when administered in very small doses, may be no more effective than placebo, though the data is conflicting. One meta-analysis of 107 homeopathy trials, conducted at the University of Limburg in The Netherlands and published in the _British Medical Journal,_ suggested a trend toward clinical efficacy, implying that homeopathy may be more effective than placebo and deserves further study.[17] However, a larger, more carefully designed meta-analysis of the data, published in the _Lancet,_ evaluated 110 homoeopathy trials and 110 matched conventional-medicine trials and focused on ferreting out study biases. This study, conducted at the University of Bern in Switzerland, demonstrated little to no efficacy of homeopathy beyond placebo.[18] I would argue that perhaps it's not the homeopathic remedies that heal; it's the homeopath.

Critics challenged the results of studies like the homeopathy meta-analysis, that led the _Lancet_ to announce "the end of homeopathy" and the "growth of truth."[19] Yet I want to point out that those criticizing the study cited it as an example of conventional medicine twisting the data to discriminate against alternative medicine.[20] If we're going to use evidence-based medicine to evaluate treatments that don't easily lend themselves to such analysis, we must be open-minded in our interpretation of results that affirm healing methods we don't fully understand. Applying negative bias to this kind of data just because we can't conjure up a biochemical explanation is unscientific.

Keep in mind that many of these studies are far from perfect. The problem with the way some of them are conducted is that it's hard to blind both the patient and the practitioner. Though some sham acupuncture studies use dummy "needles" that are able to fake out even the acupuncturist, others blind the patient only.

This fudges things up. Studies demonstrate that when clinicians know which treatment patients are getting, they inadvertently communicate this nonverbally to the patient, which is why most conventional medical trials are double-blinded, so both the researcher and the patient are in the dark about whether they're being treated with a placebo. This distinction makes clinical research into many CAM treatments fraught with bias.

The Real Goal of Treatment

Let's not get sidetracked by poor data here. Although scientists may not be able to physiologically explain the science of many CAM treatments, is this really necessary when we already have a biochemical explanation for such treatments? We know that lying on an exam table with a caring practitioner in a relaxing environment focused on the intention of healing may abort the stress responses so many of us walk around with on a daily basis, especially when we're sick. We also know that eliciting relaxation responses is known to induce positive hormonal changes and return the body to its natural state of homeostasis, which can induce self-repair of the body. Need we know more?

In conventional medical wisdom, we call anything that doesn't outperform placebo "quackery." But haven't we lost sight of the real goal? I suggest we reconsider our evaluation standards regarding the efficacy of medical treatments. If the patient is getting better, does it really matter whether the treatment is better than placebo? Is resolution of symptoms and cure of disease not the ultimate goal? Does it really matter how we achieve such a goal?

I know it's a radical concept. But I'm not the only one considering such notions.

In an editorial in the *British Medical Journal,* Yale professor Dr. David Spiegel chided skeptics for implying that, if most of the benefit of CAM therapies comes from the placebo effect, they should be consigned to the realm of quackery. He posed this question: "Is it possible that the alternative medical community has tended historically to understand something important about the experience of illness and the ritual of doctor–patient interactions that the rest of medicine might do well to hear?"[21]

The Placebo Effect in Psychotherapy

It's not just CAM treatments whose positive effects may stem more from positive belief, nurturing care, and the relaxation responses they induce than from the treatment itself. Studies show that psychotherapy may benefit patients in the same way. Certainly, data supports the notion that those getting psychotherapy fare better than those not getting it.[22] But is it really the psychotherapy, or could it be that psychotherapy induces relaxation responses due to the combination of the patient's positive belief and the loving support of a caring therapist? Are the mind and body not more likely to heal when relaxed?

In a landmark experiment conducted at Vanderbilt University and published in the *Archives of General Psychiatry,* highly experienced psychotherapists treated 15 college students who suffered from anxiety and depression, while a comparable patient group was treated by college professors who were not therapists. Patients treated by the unskilled professors showed as much improvement as patients treated by the professional therapists.[23]

Medical anthropologist Dr. Arthur Kleinman believes that attributing psychotherapy's successes to the placebo effect need not dismiss its benefits. He sees it as more of a complement. "Psychotherapy may very well be a way of maximizing placebo responses . . . but if so, it should be applauded, rather than condemned, for exploiting a useful therapeutic process which is underutilized in general health care."[24]

The Placebo Effect in Faith Healing

Though there is less clinical data in the arena of faith healing, we might argue that the same dynamic could be at play with faith healers. Think about it. People come from far and wide to be in the presence of someone they *believe* will heal them. Add to that other people in need of healing who have made a pilgrimage and who share the same positive belief. Throw in rituals and practices that reinforce the belief—the loving hug, the laying on of hands, the meditation, the herbs, the holy water—and you've got a recipe for elicitation of relaxation responses and self-healing that scientists would dub "the mega-placebo effect."[25]

Let's look at the healing waters of Lourdes as an example of this mega-placebo effect. Lourdes offers the perfect opportunity for self-healing. People set out on a pilgrimage and are often exhausted when they arrive, meaning they're mentally in a state of increased receptivity. The shrine at Lourdes involves multiple sacred symbols of healing and many opportunities for healing rituals, as well as the company of other pilgrims who have made the journey. Collectively, those who go are often infected with contagious emotion and collective hope. This alone—the belief that the healing waters will cure disease—may be enough to activate the relaxation responses that are necessary for the body to heal itself.

The Catholic Church is aware of this and has worked hard to rule out any healings that might be deemed "hysteria." Their aim is to make sure the cures are actual miracles of a divine nature, rather than the result of self-healing caused by the power of the mind. To ensure this, the Church employs physicians to verify whether a spontaneous healing "counts" as a true "sign of God." Since 1858, only 68 have met their stringent criteria.

In 1962, Vittorio Micheli was admitted to a Verona hospital with a large cancerous tumor on his left hip. Within ten months, his hip had almost completely disintegrated, leaving his bone floating in a mass of soft tissue that required a cast to keep his leg attached. As a last resort, he took a trip to Lourdes, where he bathed several times. Each time, he described a feeling of heat moving through his body. Over the next month, he experienced renewed energy, and his doctors repeated his X-rays, finding a much smaller tumor mass. The doctors were so intrigued that they documented every step of his recovery. Soon afterward, Micheli's tumor disappeared, and the bone began regenerating. Within two months, he was walking again.[26]

Anna Santaniello's miracle, the second-to-last one recorded at Lourdes, occurred after she had developed severe heart disease following acute rheumatic arthritis. She suffered from severe shortness of breath, as well as Bouillaud's disease, which made it difficult for her to speak and impossible for her to walk. She also had severe asthma attacks, cyanosis (blueness caused by lack of oxygen) of her face and lips, and lower limb swelling. After volunteers lowered her into the healing waters, her symptoms disappeared, and a doctor confirmed her cure.

Most recently, in March of 2011, 56-year-old Serge François was pronounced the latest miracle. After complications of a herniated disc left him with almost no mobility in his left leg, he made a pilgrimage to the sacred shrine in 2002 and experienced a rapid increase in mobility. He's still doing well ten years later.

In *Anatomy of an Illness*, Norman Cousins wrote, "The vaunted 'miracle cures' that abound in the literature of all the great religions . . . all say something about the ability of the patient, properly motivated and stimulated, to participate actively in extraordinary reversals of disease and disability."

Reclaiming the Heart of Medicine

As health-care providers, we are blessed with a sacred opportunity. We have the power to encourage relaxation responses in our patients and, in so doing, be part of the healing process in more ways than just drugs or surgeries. In my opinion, if we fail to optimize the self-healing mechanisms of our patients, we do them—and ourselves—a huge disservice. And if we step up to the plate and do our job well, our role in the healing process may mean the difference between life and death for the patient.

I often joke that I practice love, with a little medicine on the side. Yet, all too often, technological advances have so distanced us from our patients that the love seems to have gotten lost in the process. Whereas a physician used to do house calls, sit at the bedside, and touch the patient, we now offer 13-minute patient visits in a sterile white room where lab tests may take the place of a thorough patient history and radiological studies may even replace the hands-on physical exam. Without the healing power of listening, loving touch, nurturing care, and healing intention, what are we offering patients beyond straight technology?

When you're facing a health crisis, make sure you find the nurturing care you need. It's not enough to seek out the best surgeon or the most famous university doctor who specializes in your specific illness. Though specialized skills certainly come in handy, if you want to optimize your body's chance of cure, you'll also want to ensure that your health-care providers genuinely care. You may need more than just one person as you navigate the course of your treatment. You may need a whole team believing in you, offering you tools from their various toolboxes, and helping you make the body ripe for miracles. As you gather your team, you'll also need the members of that team to cooperate with one another.

Acupuncturist Susan Fox calls such a team of collaborative practitioners "the healing round table." The healing round table is a collaborative process in which all health-care practitioners involved in the care of the patient are equal players whose opinions matter. At the healing round table, the patient, not the doctor, presides as the utmost authority. While physicians might be invited to the healing round table, the invitation to be present does not grant doctors the right to give orders, negate the advice of others, disrespect others at the table, or, most importantly, disregard the patient's wishes.

While I understand the need to have a physician calling out orders during a trauma situation in the emergency room, the same does not apply to those caring for someone with a chronic illness. I once heard a respected physician (albeit a tired one) say to a brilliant nurse, "Let's play a little game. I'll play doctor. You play nurse. I'll give the orders, and you *follow them.*" This kind of dynamic serves neither the health-care provider nor the patient.

I've also heard doctors ridicule patients for seeking out alternative or homeopathic treatments, disrespecting both the patient and the CAM practitioner. These kinds of adversarial relationships trouble me deeply, because they speak to a much greater dysfunction within our health-care system. This dictatorial, condescending, hierarchical mind-set is more militaristic than the way I believe health-care systems should be. And while doctors in the trenches may feel they are at war against disease, replicating warlike methods of communication within hospitals and patient exam rooms doesn't help people heal. It only triggers stress responses. Health care functions much more effectively when teams work as a unit committed to serving the patient first and foremost, without ego, competition, and unnecessary power plays.

In my online community, I've been recruiting health-care revolutionaries—health-care providers and patients who are committed to bringing the *care* back to health care. If you're nodding your head and wondering where the rest of us are, don't despair. We're here, an increasingly organized and vocal population of change agents who know we must reclaim the heart of medicine and are committed to seeing change happen. Keep the faith. We need you now more than ever.

As mind-body medicine pioneer Dr. Larry Dossey wrote to me, "We really do constitute a kind of parallel medical world that exists alongside the conventional kind. We focus on what [the conventional world] knows, and we honor it, but more besides: spirituality, meaning, purpose, consciousness, compassion, empathy, love . . . And guess what? We are going to win the competition. It's really only a matter of time. But we need to dance as fast as we can, because time is not on our side. The urgency is real. So welcome to the dance!"

The time is now. Are you ready?

PART TWO

TREAT
YOUR
MIND

Chapter 4

REDEFINING HEALTH

"The great majority of us are required to live a life of constant,

systematic duplicity. Your health is bound to be affected if, day

after day, you say the opposite of what you feel, if you grovel

before what you dislike and rejoice at what brings you nothing

but misfortune. Our nervous system isn't just a fiction, it's part of

our physical body, and our soul exists in space and is inside us, like

teeth in our mouth. It can't be forever violated with impunity."

— BORIS PASTERNAK, DOCTOR ZHIVAGO

After researching the placebo and nocebo effects, I felt very comfortable authoritatively stating that the body is designed to repair itself and that positive belief, nurturing care, and the relaxation responses they induce set the stage for the body to heal itself. But are positive belief and nurturing care really enough to cure the body a decent percentage of the time? I had a sneaking suspicion it just wasn't that simple.

What about the woman who believes she will get well and finds an awesome doctor but lives with a man who cheats on her and abuses her?

What about the sick person who works 12-hour days in a demeaning job that requires he sell out his integrity in order to bring home a paycheck? What about the person who smokes, drinks, eats pasta and pepperoni pizza, and lives to be 100 because his life is so full of love, vitality, and purpose that he doesn't want to leave it? I had a sneaking suspicion that there is a lot more to optimal health than we think.

Take the health nut, for example. When people are doing everything "right" when it comes to healthy behaviors—eating their organic veggies, avoiding meat, dairy, gluten, and processed foods, exercising daily, sleeping well, avoiding addictions, seeing functional medicine doctors so they can optimize the biochemistry of the body, and so forth, we should expect them to live long, prosperous lives and die of old age while sleeping peacefully, right? So why is it that so many health nuts are sicker than others who pig out on barbecue, guzzle beer, sleep five hours a night, and veg out on the sofa in front of the boob tube?

If some health nuts are just as likely to get sick as some couch potatoes, I had to conclude that something was wrong with our definition of what constitutes a healthy lifestyle. Clearly, such healthy behaviors are a huge part of an optimally healthy life. I consider myself one of those health nuts. I drink my green juice, take my vitamins, hike and practice yoga daily, sleep well, see a functional medicine doctor, and take measures to avoid toxins that can harm me.

And yet I have come to believe that the purely physical, biochemical realm of illness—the part you can diagnose on laboratory tests, see on radiologic studies, and explain in petri dishes under microscopes, the part that benefits from diet, exercise, avoidance of toxins, and functional medicine's positive effects on the body—is only part of the equation. It's a big part, mind you, but not the whole shebang. My experience with patients (as well as my personal experience, which I'll delve into in Chapter 9) has led me to believe that whether patients get sick or stay healthy, whether they manage to heal themselves or stay sick, may have even more to do with everything else that's going on in the patient's life than with any "healthy" thing they do.

On-the-Job Training

This inkling I had about what predisposes the body to get well and what really makes us sick became clearer while I was working in an integrative medicine practice in Marin County. After leaving my conventional medicine practice, I joined a lovely group of doctors and other health-care practitioners committed to helping patients optimize their health. I was so grateful to have a whole hour with my new patients, and unlike my old practice, it gave me the opportunity to dig deep into what really predisposed my patients to illness and what really made them healthy.

When I joined the new practice, I was in awe of my new patients. They were the most health-conscious people I've ever had the privilege to serve. Many who came to the center drank their daily green juice, ate a vegan diet, worked out with personal trainers, slept eight hours a night, took a handful of vitamins and other health supplements every morning, spent a fortune on seeing CAM healers, and mindfully followed their doctors' orders religiously. This regimen worked wonders for some. They were pinnacles of health with glowing skin and gorgeous bodies and life force emanating through their pores.

But some of them were sicker than ever. I was baffled! From everything I had learned in medical school, these people should have been in perfect health. So why were so many "healthy" patients suffering?

In my attempts to help these patients, I ran batteries of tests, including specialized tests conventional doctors don't usually order, and occasionally I'd pick up something surprising that, when treated, resulted in complete resolution of the patient's symptoms. These patients thought I was a superhero. One simple hormone replacement, for example, would transform their life.

But with this subset of patients—the ones who lived healthy lives and still experienced boatloads of symptoms—more often than not, I'd find nothing and wind up shrugging my shoulders. I couldn't find a biochemical explanation for why these patients didn't feel vital. I felt like a failure as a healer, but I knew in my heart it wasn't my fault. I wasn't forgetting to order some critical test. I hadn't failed to refer them to the right specialist. The answer resided elsewhere. There was still a big missing piece of the healing puzzle. I just couldn't figure out what it was.

By this time I was really curious and really motivated to solve the puzzle of why these "healthy" patients were so sick. Instead of focusing exclusively on health behaviors, past medical history, and other traditional questions, I started asking my patients to tell me about their lives. Because we had the luxury of an hour to spend together, I could sit and listen. And what they started telling me changed how I viewed the whole notion of health.

That's when I got inspired to change my patient-intake form. Instead of limiting my questions to the patient's past medical history, past surgical history, family history, medications, and history of substance use, the way I had been taught to do in medical school, I added a laundry list of questions to my intake form about the rest of the patient's life. What I learned from these questions amazed me.

A Radical New Kind of Patient Intake

I started digging deep into the personal lives of my patients, asking questions most doctors had never thought of. Is anything keeping you from being the most authentic, vital *you?* If so, what is holding you back? What do you love and celebrate about yourself? What's missing from your life? What do you appreciate about your life? Are you in a romantic relationship? If so, are you happy? If not, do you wish you were?

Are you fulfilled at work? Do you feel like you're in touch with your life purpose? Do you feel sexually satisfied, either with a partner or by yourself? Do you express yourself creatively? If so, how? If not, do you feel creatively thwarted, like there's something within you dying to come out? Do you feel financially healthy or is money a stressor in your life?

If your fairy godmother could change one thing about your life, what would you wish for? What rules do you follow that you wish you could break?

I discovered that my patients' answers often gave me more insight into why they might be sick than any lab test, medical record review, or X-ray exam could. The diagnosis was often crystal clear in a way I previously had missed because I wasn't asking the right questions.

I came to see that these patients were unhealthy, not because of bad genes or poor health habits or rotten luck, but because they were gut-wrenchingly lonely or miserable in their bad relationships, stressed about work, freaked out about their finances, or profoundly depressed. Most, when I asked on my intake form "What's missing from your life?" wrote a long list. And when I asked the same question in person, the majority of these patients wept. Something was going on that had nothing to do with vegetables or exercise or vitamins.

On the flip side, I had other patients who ate poorly, exercised rarely, forgot to take their supplements, and enjoyed seemingly perfect health. When I read their intake forms, they revealed that their lives were filled with love, fun, meaningful work, financial abundance, creative expression, sexual pleasure, spiritual connection, and other traits that differentiated them from the sick health enthusiasts. They were, in essence, happy. And even though they didn't take the best care of their bodies, their bodies responded with good health.

That's when I began asking my patients two mother-lode questions. *"What do you think might lie at the root of your illness?"* And most important, *"What does your body need in order to heal?"*

When I first started popping these questions, I assumed people would tell me that the root cause of their illness was a hormone imbalance or an unhealthy diet. I thought they might share treatment intuitions with me. Things like "I think I'll choose craniosacral therapy over physical therapy" or "I'm gonna wait on that cholesterol drug and try changing my diet instead."

Occasionally, patients answered with insights into conventional health-related modifications they felt they needed to make—things like "I really need an antidepressant" or "Antibiotics should do the trick" or "I need to lose 20 pounds" or "I really need to get my hormones balanced."

But more often than not, when I asked, "What do you think might lie at the root of your illness?" my patients said things like these: "I give until I'm depleted." "I'm miserable in my marriage." "I absolutely hate my job." "I need more 'me' time." "I'm so lonely I cry myself to sleep every night." "I'm out of touch with my life purpose." "I don't feel God anymore." "I hate myself so much I can't look at myself in the mirror." "I'm avoiding facing the truth." "I can't forgive myself for what I've done." "I'm living a lie and I feel like a total fraud."

And when I asked my patients, "What does your body need in order to heal?" my patients shocked me with their answers. "I have to quit my job." "It's time to finally come out of the closet to my parents." "I must divorce my spouse." "I have to finish my novel." "I need to hire a nanny." "I'm so lonely, I need to make more friends." "I need to meditate every day." "I have to tell my husband I'm having an affair." "I need to forgive myself." "I need to love myself." "I need to stop being such a pessimist."

Whoa . . .

While many patients simply weren't ready to do what they knew their intuition told them their bodies needed, my bravest patients listened to the quiet voice within and made radical changes. Some quit their jobs. Others left their marriages. Some moved to new cities. Others finally pursued long-suppressed dreams.

The results these patients achieved were astonishing. Sometimes, a laundry list of illnesses would disappear, often very quickly. My patients were healing themselves after years of medical therapies had proven useless. I was in awe.

A Story of Self-Healing

Marla was the stereotypical Marin County resident. She ate a vegetarian diet, hiked and practiced yoga, competed in triathlons, took dozens of supplements her naturopath had given her, and avoided alcohol, smoking, and using any illegal drugs.

But she had a medical chart two feet thick and suffered from four different chronic health conditions.

Marla heard from some friends that my practice wasn't your usual medical practice, so she scheduled an appointment with me to see if I could figure out why she was still sick in spite of all of her efforts to get well. From reading the new patient intake probing into Marla's personal life, I found out that Marla was miserable. She was in a physically and mentally abusive marriage and hadn't had sex in two years. She felt creatively thwarted because her husband didn't support her passion for art, and she was so busy at work and training for races, she didn't make time to paint. Plus, she was exhausted from caring for her aging, sick mother, who lived in her home.

After I finished reading her form, I knew that Marla's body was never going to get well until she healed these other aspects of her life. With all those negative emotions filling her mind and all those stress hormones coursing through her body, no vegetable, supplement, exercise program, or drug was going to be strong enough to counteract the harmful health effects of chronic stress responses on her body.

After sharing with Marla my thoughts about the real reason her body was suffering, I asked her the big question. "What does your body need in order to heal?"

Marla said, "I need to move to Santa Fe."

"Why Santa Fe?" I asked.

Marla said, "I have a vacation home in Santa Fe, and whenever I go there, *all of my symptoms disappear.*"

Perhaps there was a biochemical explanation for this. Maybe she had some chemical sensitivity to something in her Mill Valley house. Maybe she was allergic to something that grew in the Bay Area but not in Santa Fe. Perhaps the weather or the food or some other environmental factor could explain such a dramatic difference.

But I doubted it, so I encouraged Marla to listen to the wisdom of her body and her intuition.

A year later, I got a call from Marla telling me she had moved to Santa Fe. In order to make such a drastic move, she sold her company and helped her mother establish herself in a wonderful retirement community close to Santa Fe, where she would be able to visit her on weekends. She also filed for divorce from her husband. And once Marla got to Santa Fe, she enrolled in art school. She had since fallen in love with a new man and met a whole new group of artist friends, and she enjoyed hiking, biking, and skiing in the mountains outside of Santa Fe.

Most important, she told me, all of her symptoms had disappeared, as if by magic, within three months of her move.

How Your Lifestyle Affects Your Body

Marla's health conditions were not cured by a drug, supplement, or surgery, but by reducing the stress in her life, relaxing her mind and body, following a dream, finding love, and filling her body with health-inducing hormones while ridding her body of harmful stress hormones. Such changes resulted in measurable physiological changes in her body.

And it wasn't just Marla. I witnessed similar transformations in dozens of patients. I finally realized that the medical establishment's nearly exclusive focus on the biochemistry of the patient's body, often to the exclusion of the health of the patient's mind, was doing our patients a grave disservice.

My experience with my Marin County patients fueled the next phase of my research into what leads to optimal health and longevity. With the same passion that sent me to the library in search of proof that the mind can heal the body, I returned to medical literature to search for what else, beyond the traditional health-inducing behaviors I was taught about in medical school, affects the health of the body via the health of the mind.

My theory—that the lifestyle choices you make can result in physiological changes in the body—extended to the people you interact with in your personal and professional life, how much creative freedom you experience, how spiritually connected you feel, your relationship with money, and how happy you are. People who make happy, healthy life choices, such as finding a loving, supportive life partner, having close relationships with friends and family, and engaging in work they love, lead lives full of positivity, which optimize the relaxation response, counteract the stress response, and lead to better health.

We all know stress is bad for us in a vague, what-do-you-expect-me-to-do-about-it sort of way. But after my initial research, I now understood the clear link between the stress the mind experiences and the way the body breaks down. I observed how emotional stressors like loneliness, frustration at work, anger about a past trauma, money worries, and fear could result in illness.

Had other scientists studied these kinds of links? Was there any proof to support the idea that good relationships lead to better health or work stress leads to sickness? It was time to go back to the journals.

I set out on a mission to prove that each facet of how you live your life affects the health of your mind and, with it, the health of your body. I predicted that, in order to live a vital life, prevent disease, or optimize the chance for disease remission, you would need:

- **Healthy relationships,** including a strong network of family, friends, loved ones, and colleagues

- **A healthy, meaningful way to spend your days,** whether you work outside the home or in it

- **A healthy, fully expressed creative life** that allows your soul to sing its song

- **A healthy spiritual life,** including a sense of connection to the sacred in life

- **A healthy sexual life** that allows you the freedom to express your erotic self and explore fantasies

- **A healthy financial life,** free of undue financial stress, which ensures that the essential needs of your body are met

- **A healthy environment,** free of toxins, natural-disaster hazards, radiation, and other unhealthy factors that threaten the health of the body

- **A healthy mental and emotional life,** characterized by optimism and happiness and free of fear, anxiety, depression, and other mental-health ailments

- **A healthy lifestyle that supports the physical health of the body,** such as good nutrition, regular exercise, adequate sleep, and avoidance of unhealthy addictions

The scientific evidence I uncovered proves my theory right. Each of these aspects of your life—your relationships, your work, your creative outflow, your spiritual life, your sex life, and so forth—has the power to either stress you or relax you. A healthy relationship elicits relaxation responses in the body. An unhealthy one flips on the stress response. A healthy spiritual life elicits positive emotions like joy, hope, and a sense of oneness, and the relaxation response turns on. An unhealthy spiritual life, one in which you feel judged by your spiritual community, fear punishment by a vindictive deity, or are threatened with negative outcomes like going to hell, is bound to trigger stress responses.

It's not enough to focus solely on the body without taking into account the health of the mind. Promoting health of the body without encouraging health of the mind is an exercise in futility. Not until we realize that our bodies are mirrors of our interpersonal, spiritual, professional, sexual, creative, financial, environmental, mental, and emotional health will we truly heal. In fact, the scientific data suggests that, at least in some instances, the health of the mind is equally, if not more, important to the health of the body. The body doesn't fuel how we live our lives. Instead, it is a mirror of how we live our lives. The body is a reflection of the sum of our life experiences.

Consider the patient with pelvic pain whose pain only appears when her abusive, controlling boss walks into her office. She goes to the gynecologist, who diagnoses her with endometriosis and suggests a surgical treatment, as well as a referral to a urologist. So she visits the urologist, who puts a camera into her bladder and diagnoses her with interstitial cystitis but suggests she see a gastroenterologist, just to be certain. Then she sees a gastroenterologist who sticks a scope up her butt and slaps her with the label of irritable bowel syndrome.

Yet nobody ever talks to her about the fact that her pain only comes when her boss is in the room. Nobody suggests that perhaps the stress of her job and her dysfunctional relationship with her boss is manifesting as physical symptoms because of repetitive stress responses in the body. Perhaps, rather than drugs or surgery, what she needs is a new job, so that she can heal her negative thoughts, allowing her body to repair itself.

Sick Versus Well

If health of the body requires health of the mind, what shall we call this kind of health? Our health-care system doesn't even have language to describe this expanded kind of health. The common definition of the word "health" doesn't take into account whether you're fulfilled at work or happy in your marriage or surrounded by a network of people who love you.

In medical school, I was taught that there are two kinds of people—sick people and well people. We all know who sick people are. They have something wrong on physical examination. They have abnormal laboratory and radiologic tests and are considered diseased or ill. They wind up taking medications, and if doctors manage to keep them from landing flat on their backs in hospitals—or even worse, dying—we breathe a sigh of relief.

If we go one step further and help them make physical lifestyle modifications that benefit the body, like diet modification or smoking cessation, and these changes cause them to feel less sick, we pat ourselves on the back and consider our jobs well done.

Well people, on the other hand, have normal physical exams, normal laboratory and radiologic results, and are generally free of disease. If they have diseases, we've controlled them with medication, dietary changes, exercise, weight loss, or whatever is working to keep them "well."

As health-care providers, we aim to prevent well people from becoming sick people, and fortunately, greater awareness of preventive health has helped make that goal a reality. Public health education about wellness-inducing behaviors, such as good nutrition, regular exercise, smoking cessation, weight control, vaccination, and cancer screening, have contributed to the wellness of the general population.

And yet, while medical technology is advancing at a rapid-fire pace and our understanding of what prevents disease continues to grow, our society is increasingly obese, hypertensive, and diabetic, suffering from heart attacks, strokes, and cancers, or doped up on drugs for anxiety, depression, and bipolar disorder.

There's another category of patients who lie somewhere in between sick people and well people. They're not technically sick but they're not exactly well either. Their blood tests come back normal. Their vital signs are stable. They're granted clean bills of health on their physicals. And yet, they don't feel vital. There's an epidemic of patients like this out there.

People suffering from this epidemic come to the doctor feeling fatigued. They feel depressed and anxious. They toss and turn at night. They suffer from decreased libido. They gain weight. They numb out with a variety of addictions. And they complain of vague physical symptoms, such as muscle aches, back and neck pain, gastrointestinal disturbances, headaches, chest tightness, and dizziness.

Suspecting something is terribly wrong, patients suffering from the epidemic go to the doctor knowing something must be wrong. The doctor runs a series of tests and winds up pronouncing the patient "well." Only the patient doesn't *feel* well.

Because doctors cannot find a biochemical explanation for the symptoms these patients experience, we tend to treat them with antidepressants and other catch-all drugs that fail to address the root cause of the issues, and the patient often fails to experience relief. So the patient goes to another doctor and starts the whole process over again because something is clearly wrong. And they're right. Something is wrong. But it's not what they think.

Many of these patients who are technically well but feel sick are suffering from the physiological consequences of repetitive stress responses that progressively break down the body. Unless the underlying stress is relieved, these patients often become genuinely sick. But the medical establishment doesn't seem to recognize this. Instead, they suggest that the physical symptoms are "all in your head." And they're sort of right. It starts in your head, and then it translates into the body.

The Physiology of Emotion

So how exactly does a thought or a feeling translate into physical effects all over the body?

You start with a thought or a feeling—take fear, for example. A doctor tells you that you have only three months to live. Or someone injects you with something they warn you will have unpleasant side effects. Or maybe it's not even that dramatic. Maybe you're afraid your wife is going to leave you or your boss is going to fire you or you won't be able to pay the bills or your dream won't come true or everybody will reject you because you're unlovable.

Your thoughts are powerful. Your conscious mind—which resides in the forebrain—knows you're frightened. But your lizard brain—the area near your brainstem that houses the hypothalamus—can't tell the difference between an abstract fear thought and a real live survival threat. Your lizard brain thinks you're about to die, and this stimulates the stress response, setting off the fight-or-flight mechanisms, activating the HPA axis, flipping on the sympathetic nervous system, shutting down your immune system, and getting you ready to run away from danger.

When your body is in the middle of a stress response, your body's self-maintenance and self-repair functions come to a screeching halt. These stress responses were meant to be triggered only very rarely. The healthy body is supposed to be in a relaxed state of physiological rest most of the time. If you're a caveman living in a happy tribe of people, you would only be expected to run from a cave bear once in a blue moon. The rest of the time, you'd be gathering berries, hanging around the campfire, and making little cavebabies.

Of course, our caveman ancestors didn't live very long because of real and present dangers they faced every day, dangers we're largely protected from because of modern luxuries like ample shelter and food. But modern life has its own perils. The stressors of daily life—things like loneliness, unhappy relationships, work stress, financial stress, anxiety, and depression—result in forebrain thoughts and feelings that repetitively trigger the hypothalamus to elicit stress responses. The mind knows it's just a feeling, but the lizard brain thinks you're under attack.

Feelings like fear, anxiety, anger, frustration, resentment, and other negative emotions trigger the HPA axis.[1] Whether or not your body is in danger, your mind believes you are, so your hypothalamus is activated and releases corticotrophin-releasing factor (CRF) into the nervous system. CRF responds by stimulating the pituitary gland, causing it to secrete prolactin, growth hormone, and adrenocorticotropic hormone

(ACTH), which stimulate the adrenal gland and cause it to release corti-sol, which in turn is responsible for helping the body maintain homeo-stasis when the brain signals a threat.

When the hypothalamus is activated, it also turns on the sympa-thetic nervous system (the fight-or-flight response), causing the adrenal glands to release epinephrine and norepinephrine, which increase pulse and blood pressure and affect other physiological responses. The secre-tion of these hormones leads to a variety of metabolic changes all over the body.

Blood vessels traveling to the gastrointestinal tract, hands, and feet constrict, while vessels traveling to the heart, large muscle groups, and brain dilate, preferentially shunting blood to the organs that will help you escape in an emergency. Your pupils dilate so more light can get in. Metabolism speeds up in order to jolt you with a boost of energy by breaking down fat stores and liberating glucose into the bloodstream. Your respiratory rate increases and your bronchi dilate, allowing more oxygen in, and your muscles become tense and ready to sprint away from the perceived threat.

Stomach acid increases and digestive enzymes decrease, often leading to esophageal contractions, diarrhea, or constipation. Corti-sol suppresses your immune system to reduce the inflammation that would accompany any wounds the attack might inflict. Reproduction gets shut off—sex is a luxury when there's danger!

Basically, your body ignores sleeping, digesting, and reproducing, and instead focuses on running, breathing, thinking, and delivering oxygen and energy in order to keep you safe. When your body is fac-ing a physical threat, these changes help you fight or flee the threat. But when the threat exists only in your mind, the body doesn't realize that there is no bodily threat, and over time, when this stress response is repetitively triggered, nature's biological response winds up actually doing more harm than good.

As a result, the body can't relax and repair what inevitably gets ill if not maintained by self-repair mechanisms. Organs get damaged. The cancer cells we naturally make every day, which usually get blast-ed away by the immune system, are allowed to proliferate. The effects of chronic wear and tear on the human body take their toll, and we wind up sick.

But it doesn't have to be this way. The body knows how to relax with the counterbalancing relaxation response Herbert Benson described (see Chapter 8). When the conscious forebrain thinks positive thoughts and feels things like love, connection, intimacy, pleasure, and hope, the hypothalamus stops triggering the stress responses. When you feel optimistic and hopeful, loved and supported, in the flow in your professional or creative life, spiritually nourished, or sexually connected to another person, the relaxation response takes the place of the stress response.

The sympathetic nervous system shuts off. Cortisol and adrenaline levels drop. The parasympathetic nervous system takes over. The immune system flips back on. And the body can go about its natural self-repair process, preventing illness and taking its stab at treating disease that already exists. As a result, disease is more likely to be prevented in well people, and disease may even be treated in sick people.

Voilà! Your thoughts lead to self-healing. The mind has healed the body, and it's not some New Age metaphysical thing. It's simple physiology.

I now firmly believe that positive belief and nurturing care turn off the stress response, trigger the relaxation response, and return the body to its natural state of physiological rest so it can do what it does best—heal itself. One of the most profound ways your mind can heal your body is through the relationships in your life. We all know that love heals, but did you know that it heals not just the soul but the body? While loneliness, anger, and resentment are poison for the body, the desire for connection, intimacy, and a sense of belonging with family, lovers, and friends is hardwired in our DNA, and when these desires are fulfilled, our bodies respond with better health. When you find your tribe, feel loved, and surround yourself with the people who know your heart and accept you just the way you are, you optimize the body's capacity for self-repair and make your body ripe for miracles.

———

Chapter 5

LONELINESS POISONS THE BODY

"How we need another soul to cling to."

— SYLVIA PLATH

When you consider how "healthy" you are, you've probably been programmed to think about your diet, your exercise regimen, your vitamins, your bad habits, your genes, and whether or not you're following doctor's orders. But have you thought about whether you feel intimately supported by a community of people you care about?

Probably not. But you should.

As it turns out, loneliness can make you sicker than smoking cigarettes and being part of a supportive community can increase your life expectancy. Don't believe me? Let me take you back in time to Roseto, Pennsylvania, in 1961, a town where a community of Italian immigrants settled together in an enclave that recreated the Old Country in the New World.

Like its namesake in the mountains of southern Italy, Roseto Valfortore, the village of Roseto, Pennsylvania, clings to a forested ridge—this one in the Poconos, where a group of Italians who first set sail for the New World in 1882 came in search of a better life.

Because of its remoteness, few outsiders make their way into the village. But come with me into the village of Roseto, and let me show you around.

In the daytime, you'll find ghost-town-empty streets, because the children are all in school and the men and the women of Roseto are working long, tedious shifts at either the stone quarry or the blouse factory, trying to earn enough money to send their kids to college.

Two-story stone houses built along the main street of Garibaldi Avenue are clustered on the rocky hillside. Our Lady of Mount Carmel Church, which came to life when the inspiring and enterprising young priest Father Pasquale de Nisco took over, towers over the other buildings. De Nisco can be credited with much of the success of the town of Roseto. He encouraged the townspeople to plant crops, raise pigs, grow grapes, set up spiritual societies, and plan celebratory festivals. Soon thereafter, schools, shops, the blouse factory, and other evidence of culture sprang to life.

In the evening, you'll see the village of Roseto come alive as people return from work, strolling along the village's main street, stopping to gossip with the neighbors, and maybe sharing a glass of wine before heading home to change into dinner clothes. As the church bell rings, you'll see women gathering together in communal kitchens, preparing classic Italian feasts, while men push tables together in anticipation of the nightly ritual that gathers the community together over heaping piles of pasta, Italian sausage, meatballs fried in lard, and free-flowing vino.

As a community of new immigrants surrounded by English and Welsh neighbors who turn up their noses at the Italians, the people of Roseto in 1961 are forced to look out for one another. Multigenerational homes are the norm. Everyone goes to church together. Neighbors wander in and out of one another's kitchens regularly, and holidays are joyously celebrated together. The work ethic in the community is strong. Not only does everyone work in Roseto; they share a common mission, a life purpose that fuels their often backbreaking work. They dream of a better life for their children.

The people of Roseto take care of one another. Nobody in Roseto is left to struggle through life alone. Roseto in 1961 is living proof of the power of the clan.

This little Pennsylvania town might have gone largely unnoticed by the rest of the world had it not been brought to the attention of Dr.

Stewart Wolf, a professor at the University of Oklahoma School of Medicine, who bought a summer home in the Poconos, not far away.

One summer, Dr. Wolf was asked to speak to the local medical society, and after the talk, one of the local docs invited him to go out for a drink. Over a couple of beers, the local doc mused about how strange it was that heart disease seemed far less prevalent in the little town of Roseto than in the adjoining town of Bangor.

Dr. Wolf was all ears. This conversation took place when heart attacks were happening in epidemic proportions, ringing in as the number-one cause of death in men under 65. Intrigued, Dr. Wolf did his homework, scanning through death certificates from Roseto and comparing them to death certificates from the surrounding towns over a period of seven years. Amazingly, the men of Bangor had heart-attack rates paralleling the national average, but the heart-attack rate in Roseto was *half* the national average. In fact, it was nearly zero for men under 65. It wasn't just heart disease, though. The death rate from all causes was 30 to 35 percent lower than average in Roseto.

This finding merited further investigation.

As Malcolm Gladwell reported in *Outliers,* John Bruhn, a sociologist hired to help investigate, recalls, "There was no suicide, no alcoholism, no drug addiction, and very little crime. They didn't have anyone on welfare. Then we looked at peptic ulcers. They didn't have any of those either. These people were dying of old age. That's it."[1]

At this point Dr. Wolf and his team were committed to figuring out why the people of Roseto were so immune to disease. Attempting to answer this question, researchers poked, prodded, examined, and interviewed two-thirds of the village's adults. Dr. Wolf initially suspected they must have some Old World dietary practice making them more immune to infection. Perhaps it was all the olive oil. So he hired 11 dieticians to follow the people of Roseto into the grocery stores and watch them cook.

But that wasn't it. Unable to afford olive oil—the healthiest option—the people of Roseto cooked with lard, and they routinely ate pizza loaded with sausage, pepperoni, salami, and eggs. In fact, a shocking 41 percent of their calories came from fat.

Further, the Italian-Americans in Roseto weren't physically fit. In fact, most smoked and remained sedentary, and many were obese. So what else might explain the disparity? Dr. Wolf suspected genetics. Because the Rosetans all originated from the same small village in Italy, Dr. Wolf suspected they might have inherited some disease-protective gene. So he tracked down other immigrants originating from Roseto Valfortore, who lived elsewhere in the United States, to see if they were as healthy as their Pennsylvania cousins.

But those who originated from the same village but were scattered about the United States were no more healthy than average. Genetics couldn't explain it.

Dr. Wolf then evaluated Roseto's geography. Perhaps it was something in their water or the quality of the hospital where they received medical care. The same kind of evaluation went on in two neighboring towns where the rates of heart disease were in line with the national average. But it wasn't the water. They shared water with the neighboring communities of Nazareth and Bangor, where people were as sick as the general population. It wasn't the hospital, which they also shared, or the climate, which was the same.

Dr. Wolf finally realized that, if it wasn't their diet or their geography or their genes or the quality of their health care, there must be something disease-protective about Roseto itself. He concluded that a supportive, tight-knit community was a better predictor of heart health than cholesterol levels or tobacco use.

Dr. Wolf completed his initial study just as the golden age of Roseto's community life began to disintegrate. While the people of Roseto slaved away in the quarry and the blouse factory, sacrificing so their children could go to college and live the American dream, the younger generation wasn't so thrilled about life in Roseto, which to them seemed immune to modernization. When the young people went off to study at college, they brought back to Roseto new ideas, new dreams, and new people. Italian-Americans started marrying non-Italians. The children strayed from the church, joined country clubs, and moved into single-family suburban houses with fences and pools.

With these changes, the multigenerational homes disbanded and the community lifestyle shifted gears from nightly celebration to more of the typical "every man for himself" philosophy that fueled the neighboring communities. The neighbors who would regularly drop in for casual visits started phoning each other to schedule appointments. The evening rituals of adults singing songs while children played with marbles and jacks turned into nights in front of the television.

In 1971, when heart attack rates in other parts of the country were dropping because of widespread adoption of healthier diets and regular exercise programs, Roseto had its first heart attack death in someone younger than 45. Over the next decade, heart-disease rates in Roseto doubled. The incidence of high blood pressure tripled. And the number of strokes increased. Sadly, by the end of the 1970s, the number of fatal heart attacks in Roseto had increased to the national average.

As it turns out, human beings nourish one another, even more than spaghetti, and the health of the body reflects this. Dr. Wolf, who continued to study the community of Roseto for many years, concluded that an isolated individual may become easily overwhelmed by the challenges of everyday life, and this kind of overwhelm can trigger stress responses in the body. An individual surrounded by a supportive community, however, relaxes. This kind of relaxation translates into positive effects on the body's physiology, leading to disease prevention and, sometimes, disease remission.

Supportive Community as Preventive Medicine

It may seem obvious to you that healthy relationships are good for the body. You might be thinking, "Duh! No news flash here."

But when's the last time your doctor asked you whether your toxic ex-husband might be causing your fibromyalgia, or your abusive mother's tongue-lashings could be predisposing you to heart disease? When was the last time you asked *yourself* that?

In the rest of this chapter, I'll show how social ties and healthy relationships, including romantic relationships, healthy sexuality, and the support of a spiritual community, affect not just your happiness, but your physiology.

The reality is that loneliness causes stress, while loving community relaxes you. The effects of stress and relaxation don't just affect the mind; they affect the body. When you lack supportive community and feel you must handle life alone, the daily overwhelm may trigger anxiety, which the brain perceives as a threat. Such overwhelm adversely affects everything from blood pressure to kidney function. The negative consequences of overwhelm and stress can be mitigated, as it turns out, when you are nurtured by friends, relatives, and neighbors who care. In fact, this factor alone may affect your body more profoundly than what you eat, how much you drink, whether or not you smoke, or how much you exercise.[2]

The Effect of Community on Life Expectancy

When you think about behaviors that will increase your life expectancy, you probably think about giving up booze, taking a daily walk, taking your vitamins, cutting back on processed foods, and wearing your seat belt more than you think about joining a club, inviting friends over for dinner, or getting a cool roommate. But perhaps it's time to rethink your preventive health strategy and start treating yourself with the medicine of positive relationships.

It's not just Roseto that shows that a supportive community impacts health. Similar studies in Peru, Israel, Borneo, and elsewhere have confirmed what researchers discovered in the small Pennsylvania village, that a community of loved ones may affect your health more than what you eat, how you exercise, and whether or not you have good or bad health habits.[3]

One study examining the people of Alameda County, California, found that, in every age and sex category, people with the fewest social ties were three times more likely to die over a nine-year period than those who reported the most social ties, even when you account for preexisting health conditions, socioeconomic status, smoking, alcohol consumption, obesity, race, life satisfaction, physical activity, and use of preventive health services.[4] Those with more social connections were even found to have lower rates of cancer.[5]

How much we commune with other people may prove to be as important as exercise when it comes to predicting life expectancy. A Harvard study examining the lives of almost 3,000 senior citizens found that those who gather together to go out to dinner, play cards, go on day trips, vacation with friends, go to the movies, attend sporting events, go to church, and engage in other social activities outlive their reclusive peers by an average of two and a half years. In fact, these kinds of mostly stationary social activities were found to benefit the health of the seniors as much as fitness-related activities did. The researchers concluded that social pursuits are equivalent to and independent of the merits of exercise.[6] Many more studies confirm that social ties and life expectancy are inextricably linked.[7]

The degree of social support you experience even affects the likelihood of cure if you do wind up sick. A University of California, San Francisco study published in the *Journal of Clinical Oncology* investigated the social networks of nearly 3,000 nurses with breast cancer. This study found that the women who had been socially isolated before their breast cancer diagnosis had a 66 percent higher risk of mortality from any cause and a twofold risk of breast cancer mortality. The nurses who went through cancer alone were found to be four times more likely to die from their disease than those with ten or more friends supporting their journey. In fact, the data suggests that friendships may be even more health-inducing than having a spouse. In the same study, having a spouse did not show a survival benefit—but having many friendships did.[8]

The same protective effect of a strong support network was seen in a study performed at Sahlgrenska University in Sweden and published in the *European Heart Journal,* which investigated the social lives of 741 men with heart disease over a period of 15 years and determined that those with the highest measures of what they called "social integration" were the most protected against new heart attacks.[9]

In a *New Scientist* article about the effects of loneliness on health, Dr. Charles Raison, professor of psychiatry at Emory University School of Medicine, concluded, "People who have rich social lives and warm, open relationships don't get sick and they live longer."[10]

Spiritual Community and Health

You might not consider going to church a health-inducing behavior, but it is. A study conducted by the California Public Health Foundation, which was published in the *American Journal of Public Health,* found a strong association between attendance at religious services and lower mortality over a 28-year period for 5,286 Alameda County residents.[11] Another study, conducted at the Buck Institute for Research on Aging and also published in the *American Journal of Public Health,* evaluated religious attendance and subsequent mortality over a five-year span for 1,931 elderly residents of Marin County, California. Once again, the findings found that religious service attendance had a protective effect on life expectancy.[12]

In fact, as still another study showed, if you have heart surgery and receive support and strength from your religious community, you'll be three times more likely to be alive six months later.[13]

But why is religion so good for your health? You might think it's because people who go to church are less likely to be out boozing it up, getting high, or having one-night stands. And you'd be right. Religious people tend to behave better than their nonreligious peers.[14] In fact, many religious groups, such as Mormons or Orthodox Jews, actively promote a low-stress, positive lifestyle that advocates moderation and a harmonious family life.

But that alone doesn't explain the difference. It's more than that. People who attend religious services have larger social networks. A religious community prevents isolation and fosters better health.[15] The positive effect of spiritual community on the body's health is dramatic, possibly because places of worship encourage socialization, and people who share religious beliefs tend to take care of one another the way the people of Roseto did.

Individuals who attend religious services regularly live seven and a half years longer (almost 14 years longer for African-Americans) than those who never or rarely attend religious gatherings.[16] People who are part of a spiritual community have also been shown to have lower blood pressure and reduced risk of cardiovascular disease, lower rates of depression and suicide, lower rates of substance abuse, and stronger immune systems.[17] Mormons, whose faith leads them to gather in tight-knit communities based on shared religious beliefs, have even been shown to experience 24 percent less cancer than the general population.[18]

In the Alameda County studies, researchers found that high levels of religious involvement were associated with lower rates of circulatory diseases, digestive diseases, respiratory diseases, and just about every other disease studied. In fact, the protective effect on health of weekly attendance at a religious event was so strong that it equaled the effect of smoking and regular exercise on health.[19]

There's no question that involvement in a spiritual community prevents social isolation. Like the residents of Roseto, who took care of one another and ensured that nobody was ever lonely, religious communities often offer similar communal support, and the evidence suggests that the body responds with better health. But there may be other explanations for why people who participate in spiritual communities are more likely to be healthy.

In addition to the relaxation responses induced by supportive community, faith in a higher power may also induce positive emotions, which counteract stress and contribute to the state of physiological rest necessary for the body to repair itself. People with faith in a higher power are also likely to experience better health because they are better able to find meaning in the face of loss or trauma. One study showed that religious parents who lost babies to sudden infant death syndrome were better able to cope 18 months later than nonreligious parents.[20] Religious people are also more apt to forgive, which alleviates negative emotions such as anger and resentment that trigger the stress response.[21]

While those who believe in a loving divinity are more likely to be happier and healthier than those who don't,[22] you don't have to subscribe to any particular religion or even believe in a higher power to reap the benefits of being more spiritual. Although traditional institutional religious settings offer the benefit of community linked by shared belief, you can also improve your health by being more spiritual in your own way.

Spirituality, which has been defined by social scientists as the search for the sacred, can still offer health benefits, as you acknowledge and appreciate the sacred in life—the holiness of nature, the blessing of children, the perception of your work as a calling, the body as a vessel for love in the world, the sanctity of marriage. By imbuing the ordinary with extraordinary qualities, you open yourself up to transcendence, which can elicit relaxation in the body, leading to more happiness and, subsequently, better health. Spiritual people are also happier, have better mental health, use fewer drugs and alcohol, have better coping skills, and live longer than those who don't consider themselves spiritual.[23]

Keep in mind that religion isn't all roses when it comes to the effect on your health. Like all facets of life, your spiritual life has the potential to stress you out as well as relax you. People for whom religion stirs up feelings of guilt, shame, repression, and fear of recrimination from a punishing God are more likely to experience repetitive stress responses, which result in poor health.[24] So it's not just spiritual life that can heal you, it's the *right* kind of spiritual life, one that is aligned with the truth of what is sacred *for you*.

Coupled Relationships and Health

If you don't think of marriage as a prescription for longevity or cohabitating with your lover as treatment for what ails you, it might be time to reconsider. While being part of a community has been demonstrated to improve health outcomes, the medical literature also suggests that being part of a coupled relationship benefits the body. The data shows that marriage affects not just your health, but your life expectancy.[25]

A University of California, Los Angeles study that was published in the *Journal of Epidemiology and Community Health* reviewed census data and found that those who never marry are 58 percent more likely to die at a young age than those who exchange vows.[26] Happily married people also have lower blood pressure[27] and less insomnia.[28]

Are you in love but not yet married? Don't worry. It's not just married people who benefit from the health effects of being part of a couple. A New Zealand study conducted by a team at the University of Otago, which was published in the *British Journal of Psychiatry,* examined 1,000 people and found that those in extended partnerships—regardless of whether they were married—were less likely to suffer from depression or alcohol abuse.[29]

Another study, conducted at the University of Chicago and Northwestern University and published in the journal *Stress,* investigated 500 MBA students—almost half of whom were married or in relationships. The students were instructed to play a series of economic computer games, which they believed were part of their exams. Saliva samples were taken before and after to measure hormone levels, such as the stress hormone cortisol. To create an environment of stress, each student was told that the test was a course requirement and that it would impact his or her future career placement.

Concentrations of stress hormones increased in all participants, but unpaired individuals of both sexes had higher levels of stress hormones than those who were in committed relationships. Researchers concluded: "Although marriage can be pretty stressful, it should make it easier for people to handle other stressors in their lives."[30]

While some people are happy to stay single, most people yearn for intimate connection with a romantic partner. We are biologically programmed to mate, and the positive benefits on health demonstrated by those in happily coupled relationships suggest a survival advantage in such mating that benefits the body. How do coupled relationships improve health? Most likely through the power of the mind. When you feel loved, supported, and nurtured in a relationship, your mind experiences fewer stress responses and elicits more relaxation responses, and the physiology of the body responds accordingly.

Keep in mind that merely pairing off isn't the answer. Coupled relationships can be the source of both stress and relaxation. It's not just any relationship that will benefit your health—it's the right one. When it comes to your health, you're actually better off single than in a bad relationship.[31] An unhappy marriage can harm your health, as demonstrated by an Ohio State University study published in the journal *Cancer,* which examined 100 patients with breast cancer and demonstrated that those in bad marriages fared less well than those in happy marriages.[32]

Abusive marriages also pose health risks, not just relating to injury but because of other causes of illness. Married or cohabitating women who are victims of domestic abuse are more likely to get sick.[33] So don't stay in a bad relationship just because you think it will benefit your health. The key is to foster relationships that initiate relaxation responses rather than those that trigger stress responses.

Have you lost a partner? When one-half of a couple dies, it's especially important for the surviving partner to seek support from others. One study showed that men and women who had lost a spouse from sudden, accidental death were much more likely to get sick themselves. However, if the widows and widowers confided in others close to them, they had fewer health problems and were more likely to be happy.[34]

Sexuality and Health

Another well-documented health advantage people in coupled relationships usually enjoy is sex. With all the warnings about the dangers of sex—sexually transmitted diseases, rape, sexual abuse, and the risks of pregnancy—you might not realize that sex can be good for your health. But studies show that the benefits of a healthy sexual relationship with an intimate partner improve the health of the body in remarkable ways.

Those with healthy sexual lives live longer, have a lower risk of heart disease and stroke, get less breast cancer, bolster their immune systems, sleep better, appear more youthful, enjoy improved fitness, have enhanced fertility, get relief from chronic pain, experience fewer migraines, suffer from less depression, and enjoy an improved quality of life.[35]

The evidence is mounting. Sex isn't just fun—it's good for your health! While some of the benefits of an active sex life may be attributable to the physical workout of a good romp in the hay, the positive effects of a healthy sex life on the mind—eliciting the physiological relaxation response and its counteracting effects on the stress response—may even more dramatically affect the physiology of the body.

But like all facets of how we live our lives, sex has the potential to stress you out too. If you're sexually frustrated, feeling distrustful of your partner, cheating on your spouse, losing your libido, or experiencing pain with sex, your sex life can also trigger stress responses. The key to using your sex life as a tool for preventive health and disease treatment is to ensure that it's healthy and leaves you feeling relaxed, not stressed. If your sex life is stressing you out, addressing the underlying issues coming between you and a healthy sex life is crucial.

The Physiology of Loneliness

So what is it about living in a close-knit community, gathering together with others who share your faith, being part of a coupled relationship, having lots of friends, and enjoying sexual intimacy with another person that stimulates better health?

Healthy relationships are medicine for the mind, and as we've already seen, the mind has powerful effects on the physiology of the body. So many people, especially those in the developed world, suffer from social isolation. While social isolation can sometimes be positive—a way to recharge the mind through retreats, meditation, personal time, and other nourishing, health-inducing activities—chronic social isolation can lead to loneliness, and multiple studies demonstrate that loneliness can trigger stress responses in the body, the same kind of fight-or-flight responses fear of bodily harm can elicit.

Everyone feels lonely from time to time, but for some people loneliness becomes the norm. Canadian psychologist Vello Sermat, who studies loneliness, estimates that 10 to 30 percent of people suffer from a pervasive feeling of loneliness.[36] In another study, 16 percent of people responding to a newspaper advertisement described themselves as being "lonely most or all of the time."[37] Among lonely people, 37 percent describe their health as "poor" or "very poor."[38]

As Robert Putnam put it in *Bowling Alone,* "As a rough rule of thumb, if you belong to no groups but decide to join one, you cut your risk of dying over the next year in half. If you smoke and belong to no groups, it's a toss-up statistically whether you should stop smoking or start joining. These findings are in some way heartening. It's easier to join a group than to lose weight, exercise regularly, or quit smoking."[39]

As it turns out, psychologist John Cacioppo, who has devoted his life's work to studying the effects of social isolation and loneliness on the body, agrees that curing loneliness is as good for your health as giving up smoking. According to Cacioppo, lonely people are physiologically different from people with strong social networks when it comes to cortisol-signaling genes, the inflammatory response, and the immune system.[40] Lonely people demonstrate higher diastolic blood pressure responses to stress, altered immune response, and greater cortisol responses to stress.[41]

Lonely people have also been shown to have higher rates of heart disease, breast cancer, Alzheimer's disease, and suicidal thoughts.[42] Loneliness even affects mortality rates after coronary artery bypass surgery. A Swedish study examining 1,290 patients undergoing heart surgery found that patients who agreed with the statement "I feel lonely" had significantly higher mortality rates post-operatively.[43]

In studies comparing lonely and non-lonely individuals, lonely people were found to have significantly altered cardiovascular function, including higher levels of peripheral resistance in the blood vessels, higher blood pressure, lower levels of blood-vessel-relaxing carbon monoxide, and alterations in heart rate and cardiac contractility that mimic what happens when the body is facing a threat.

Researchers also suspect that lonely individuals suffer from poor-quality sleep, and limited sleep is known to lower glucose tolerance, elevate cortisol levels, and increase fight-or-flight sympathetic nervous system activation. These effects mirror what is seen in normal aging and may explain why the body suffers in lonely individuals.[44]

Chronically lonely individuals have been found to have higher salivary cortisol levels across the course of a day, suggesting more discharges of corticotropin-releasing hormone and activation of the HPA axis, which triggers stress responses.[45] Multiple studies also demonstrate that loneliness leads to suppressed immune function, which can alter the body's ability to fight infection, mount an attack against cancer cells, and repair the body internally.[46]

Cacioppo suggests that ending loneliness is not so much about spending more time with people. He thinks it is all about altering our *attitude* toward others. Lonely people may come to view other human beings as potentially dangerous. When we feel we are in danger, harmful stress hormones and other fear chemicals are triggered. When we heal the loneliness, the body may follow.

The mind might recognize loneliness for what it is—a feeling of disconnection, of not belonging, of feeling unloved—but the lizard brain only knows one way to communicate with the rest of the body. "Houston, we have a problem!" While the mind might be able to differentiate between facing up against a wild animal on the prowl and feeling lonely, the slew of hormones the mind spews out in response to a threat is exactly the same in the body. When the mind signals the alert, your hypothalamus, pituitary gland, and adrenal glands come to life, and a surge of stress hormones, such as adrenaline, norepinephrine, and cortisol, course through your bloodstream, galloping off like Paul Revere to tell all the other organs there's a wild animal on the loose.

Normally, when the lizard brain perceives that the lion is gone, the stress-response systems reset, alerting the organs to go back to business as usual. But if you feel chronically lonely, your body may switch on the stress-response alert and leave it on, which, in time, can not only damage your health; it can shorten your life. When loneliness is known to pose as much health risk as smoking, shouldn't doctors be prescribing social support and alleviation of loneliness as part of an optimally healthy lifestyle?

All Relationships Are Not Created Equal

The scientific data supports the notion that healthy relationships affect the mind, which in turn, affects the body. But clearly, all relationships are not created equal. Many lonely individuals have chosen to be alone as a response to traumatic relationships that can harm the mind and the body. We know that childhood abuse or neglect can shorten a person's lifespan.[47] People who endure relationships characterized by conflict or hostility suffer physically and emotionally.[48] Clearly, physically abusive marriages can injure or kill you. When your clan is a street gang that engages in regular shoot-outs, your health is obviously at risk.

When your community revolves around injecting heroin together, your health would be better served by being alone.

While these examples of how the wrong relationships can harm you may seem obvious, you might be less aware of how other, more subtle types of unsupportive social ties may damage your health. You may not realize that when your church community judges you because you don't conform to social norms, your mind is likely to mount a stress response that could negatively affect your body. When your family routinely chews you a new one every time you go home to visit, Sunday afternoon family dinners might not be as beneficial to your health as they were in Roseto. When you're hanging out with the mommy crowd from your kid's school but you're feeling like it's unsafe to be authentic, your body may sense a threat.

It's old news that unhealthy relationships are bad for you. This is no shocker. You probably have relationships in your life you know are harming you, but you may not realize how they affect the physiology of the body. When you get cancer, you may not automatically leap to the conclusion that your abusive marriage could have weakened your immune system through chronic activation of the stress response. When you have a heart attack, you may not link it to your sister, who verbally beats you up every time you call, or your "friend" who cuts you down every time you see each other and gossips about you behind your back.

Although the data suggests that we need the company of other humans in order to be optimally healthy, what we really need are healthy, genuine relationships that allow us to be who we really are without judgment or criticism. Social contact simply isn't enough. If you surround yourself with people who make you feel like it isn't safe to be vulnerable, your body will manifest a stress response.

Other negative relationship dynamics, such as aggression, hate, or withdrawal of love, stimulate the stress response, whereas love, nurturing, compassion, and feelings of attachment and belonging trigger the release of hormones that induce relaxation and feelings of pleasure, such as oxytocin, dopamine, and endorphins.

In other words, be social. Avoid loneliness. Surround yourself with friends and family. But be mindful of the relationships you choose to bring into your life. Choose your inner circle wisely, and make sure, at the end of the day, you feel supported by those in your social community, rather than judged, criticized, bullied, pressured, or threatened.

As a general rule, human beings are social animals. Historically, bonding in community offered an evolutionary advantage in a world rife with threats. Deep in our souls, we long for love, belonging, and human connection. Yes, some of us are introverts and some are extroverts. Some have had our hearts broken and seek isolation as a protective mechanism from further trauma to the heart. Some have a greater need for human connection, while others find that what our minds and bodies need in order to elicit physiological relaxation are hours of solitary meditation. Ultimately, you must tap into the healing wisdom of your own intuition in order to determine what will nourish you, your mind, and your body.

It's hard to open yourself up to relationships when you feel unsafe. Opening your heart and exposing your soft underbelly feels like the last thing you want to do when your heart has been traumatized, as so many of ours have. But it's essential to open up. Shame, secrecy, and isolation are the enemies of the healing process.

The Power of Vulnerability

As a professor at the University of Houston, Brené Brown, author of *Daring Greatly* and *The Gifts of Imperfection,* studies shame, fear, and the power of vulnerability to transform shame into intimate connection with other human beings. In a viral TEDx talk "The Power of Vulnerability," as well as in her books, Brown discusses the role of shame and how it leads to social isolation. She teaches that the courage to be vulnerable, the cultivation of compassion for the imperfections of others, and the creation of healthy boundaries set the stage for healthy relationships.

In *The Gifts of Imperfection,* Brown writes, "If we want to live and love with our whole hearts, and if we want to engage with the world from a place of worthiness, we have to talk about the things that get in the way—especially shame, fear, and vulnerability." She describes shame as the fear of being unlovable and states that it exists for us all: "To feel shame is to be human."

How we shame ourselves and what we shame ourselves about varies from individual to individual but runs the gamut—body image, work, money, relationships, addictions, parenting, sex, aging, family, and more. But there's good news. If we're all capable of feeling shame, we're all also capable of what Brown calls "shame resilience"—the ability to recognize shame when it rears its ugly head, move through it in a healthy way, hang on to our sense of worthiness and authenticity, and use it to develop more courage, compassion for others who feel their own shame, and connection with others as a result.

According to Brown, the difference between guilt and shame is that guilt implies "I did something bad," while shame suggests "I am bad." While guilt is often a motivator to live with more integrity, shame is nothing but poison that gets in the way of authentic relationships. Brown recommends, instead, mustering up the courage to be vulnerable and authentic, embracing self-compassion, letting go of perfectionism, and cultivating what she calls "Wholeheartedness," the practice of living and loving with a whole heart.

In her research on shame, fear, and vulnerability, Brown found that wholehearted people live lives full of worthiness, rest, play, trust, faith, intuition, hope, authenticity, love, belonging, joy, gratitude, and creativity, while avoiding perfectionism, numbing, certainty, exhaustion, self-sufficiency, being cool, fitting in, judgment, and scarcity.[49]

Every day is an opportunity to deepen your connections to the people you value. When you let your heart feel, become resilient to shame, end your judgments of others, learn the art of forgiveness, practice being authentic, and lay bare your soul, you allow your mind to work its wonders, optimizing the body for its natural state of self-repair.

Rx for Loneliness

If you live a solitary life and have either given up trying to be more social or chosen to remain alone, you may be able to counterbalance some of the negative effects on health caused by loneliness and social isolation. In Chapter 8, I'll be teaching you some techniques you can employ at home to elicit relaxation responses and tone down stress responses.

If you're lonely and motivated to improve your health, or if you're involved in toxic relationships and need an antidote to the harm these relationships may be inflicting on your body, stay tuned. In Chapter 10, you'll have the chance to diagnose any relationship imbalances in your life and come up with an action plan for how you might relieve loneliness and enjoy the health benefits of healthy relationships.

Until then, I want you to know that the best way to alleviate loneliness is to tap into the essential nature of who you really are. Let the world see your real, authentic, beautiful fabulousness. So many of us expend so much energy trying to be someone we're not in order to fit in. In our efforts to be accepted, we lose a part of ourselves, and our health suffers as a consequence.

The truth is that people aiming to be socially acceptable are trying to hit the bull's-eye of a constantly moving target of acceptability, which means staying on top of trends, comparing yourself to others, sacrificing what you really love for what you think others love, and adhering to artificial standards of conformity. The more cool you try to be, the more isolated you'll feel. As Brené Brown said in a moving speech at the World Domination Summit hosted by author/blogger Chris Guillebeau, "The number one barrier to belonging is fitting in." It's a guaranteed recipe for loneliness. It's also a heavy price to pay, one that can leave you not only lonely but sick.

You may be tempted to seek social acceptance so you won't feel like a misfit or wind up hurt. We all want to feel loved and accepted. We long to belong. But at what price? Is it worth selling out who you are and replacing the real you with some plastic version constantly re-created to fit today's elusive acceptability factor (which you can guarantee is different than yesterday's)?

Nope.

Stripping off your masks and letting your inner radiance shine forth might not be "cool," but it allows an opportunity for deep connection. It takes real courage to be unapologetically uncool—and there's really nothing cooler in my book than people brave enough to be who they really are, even when it flies in the face of everything popular culture commands you to be. When you're brave enough to be unapologetically *you,* you become a magnet for all the others who long to be fearless enough to do the same. That, my friend, is a surefire way to alleviate loneliness.

———————————

Chapter 6

DEATH BY OVERWORK

"Unnatural work produces too much stress."

— BHAGAVAD GITA

Y ou already know that workplace hazards can harm your health. The
soldier dies in battle. The policeman gets caught in the criminal's
crosshairs. A construction worker falls from a 20-story building. A researcher experiences a biohazard accident and winds up with a rare infectious disease.

What you do during your workday can clearly affect the body. But
it affects the body not just through physical hazards. It also affects the
body through the power of the mind, which responds to what you do
during your workday by either triggering stress responses or initiating
relaxation responses. You know work has the potential to stress you out.
But you may have also experienced times at work when you're doing
what you love, you're in the flow, you feel a sense of mission and purpose, and you're grateful to be doing something that matters. Such feelings can benefit the body as much as stress responses harm it.

We all know that work stress is poisonous and can translate into
physical symptoms. Anyone who has ever gotten a migraine after a
deal went bad or stiff shoulders after the boss criticized him can attest
to that.

But has your doctor ever prescribed doing work you love as treatment for your tumor or suggested that quitting your job might cure your irritable bowel syndrome? When was the last time you diagnosed your job stress as the root cause of your stroke or credited your professional fulfillment with the spontaneous remission of your chronic disease?

Perhaps it's time for a paradigm shift.

You may not have thought much about how your work affects your health. If you're sick, you may have assumed that your illness is the result of a defective gene, poor diet, insufficient exercise, or a biochemical imbalance—and this may indeed be true. But work stress may be a contributing, even causative, factor. You might be surprised to realize that the prescription for your illness might not be a pill or surgery. It might be finding new ways to handle work stress, making changes in your current job in order to reduce anxiety, or even finding a new career.

As it turns out, you really can work yourself to death. You can also follow your bliss back to health. In Japan, there is more awareness about the effect of job stress on health. They even have a word for it—*karoshi,* which is defined as "death by overwork."

Like many of the other 7.7 million Japanese who slog their way through 60-plus-hour work weeks, Satoru Hiraoka was a good soldier, the kind who prioritized the company first and his family last, while banishing any frivolous notions like leisure time, weekends off, or vacation days. For over 28 years, Hiraoka, a middle manager at the Tsubakimoto Seiko precision bearing factory in Osaka, dutifully worked 12- to 16-hour days, often capping out at 95 hours of work each week.

This was no exaggeration. Review of Hiraoka's time cards showed that in the year prior to his untimely death, Hiraoka put in over 1,400 hours of overtime. Like the perfect employee, he never called in sick, never took a hangover day, nor skipped out on work to catch his child's school play. He was the ideal *kigyo-senchi* ("corporation soldier").[1]

Then one day, on February 23, 1988, after putting in a 15-hour day, the 48-year-old came home from work and suffered from what the doctors called "sudden cardiac insufficiency." He died instantly.

Hiraoka's death, and tens of thousands of others just like his, might have gone unnoticed had a group of Japanese occupational-medicine specialists and cardiologists not been studying the phenomenon. These doctors noticed that people who were overworked were at increased risk of dying of unexpected cardiovascular and cerebral diseases, such as heart attack and stroke. The first case had been reported in 1969, when a worker died of a stroke at the age of 29.[2]

But it wasn't until 1987 that the Japan Ministry of Labor began collecting statistics on karoshi. Since that time, Japanese officials estimate that approximately 10,000 cases of karoshi occur each year.[3] Some lawyers and scholars claim that the number of karoshi deaths in Japan equals or exceeds the number of traffic-accident fatalities each year.[4]

According to Shunichiro Tajiri, head of the Osaka-based Social Medical Study Institute, karoshi victims are typically otherwise healthy men in their 40s and 50s who are middle managers in stressful jobs that require them to work more than 12-hour days, six or seven days a week. Just before dying, most complain of varying combinations of dizziness, nausea, severe headache, and stomachache. In 95 percent of karoshi cases, death occurs within 24 hours of the onset of severe symptoms, though milder symptoms sometimes precede the severe ones.

In a *Chicago Tribune* article, Tajiri said, "In each case, the men were healthy, with no evidence of any disease. They simply worked themselves to death."

Hiraoka's widow is one of many Japanese who filed karoshi claims to receive workers' compensation benefits. But because karoshi is itself not quite a disease—it's a constellation of what are believed to be stress-induced physiological changes—and because it's often hard to prove that a victim's death is directly related to too much work stress or long hours, these benefits can be tougher to secure than those given to people who die from on-the-job accidents.[5] Nonetheless, karoshi claims are rising, and workers' compensation benefit payouts are too.

Death by Overwork in the United States

It's not just the Japanese who are working themselves to death, and it's not a new phenomenon. In June of 1863, a London newspaper reported a story entitled "Death from Simple Over-work" about a 20-year-old woman who died after working days that averaged over 16 hours a day (up to 30-hour shifts during the busy season) in a garment factory. While this might sound like the stuff of Dickensian novels, the truth is that it's happening right now in the United States, as much as it is in Japan or England.

The Information Age has transformed us into workaholics who no longer have the forced respite of snail mail and hand-delivered memos. Now, it's not just doctors who are on call 24/7. It's most of us. The advent of e-mail, cell phones, pagers, fax machines, laptops, and iPads means we are accessible almost all the time and increasingly poor employee health is reflecting it. Not that poor health stops employees from coming in to work. A study conducted by the health insurer Oxford Health Plans found that one in five Americans come to work even if they're ill, injured, or seeing a doctor that day.[6] The same sort of work obsession has about a third of employed Americans failing to use accrued vacation time, according to a survey by Expedia.com.

Similarly, about a quarter of British workers do not take all their vacation time, and in France, many don't either. The difference is that most Europeans get much more vacation time—an average of 26 days for the British and 37 for the French—compared with 14 days for the average American. Another difference is that, while 137 countries mandate paid vacation time, the United States is the only industrialized country that does not.[7]

This failure to take a break has actually been associated with early death. One study, published in *Psychosomatic Medicine* in 2000, looked at 12,000 men over nine years and found that those who failed to take annual vacations had a 21 percent higher risk of death from all causes and they were 32 percent more likely to die of a heart attack.[8]

In another study published in the *American Journal of Epidemiology,* researchers at Johns Hopkins evaluated data collected from patients in the Framingham Heart Study over a period of 20 years and found that women who vacationed once every 6 years or less often were almost eight times more likely to develop coronary heart disease or have a heart attack than women who vacationed twice a year.[9]

There's a good reason why Workaholics Anonymous is now an active 12-step program in the United States as well as in many countries.

Although most of the data on karoshi comes from Japan, the International Labour Organization released statistics showing that the United States far exceeds the Japanese when it comes to overwork. Our doctors and our government have yet to recognize karoshi as a distinct disease or award workers' compensation benefits the way the Japanese do, and because we don't track it, it's hard to say how frequently work stress manifests as death in the United States. But you can bet it affects the health of many.

Types of Job Stress

People who experience stress at work get their stress responses repetitively triggered throughout the workday. Imagine the red-faced, pot-bellied prosecuting attorney screaming at the quivering, weepy witness—like a cartoon character with steam coming out of his ears—until the attorney keels over in the middle of the courtroom with a heart attack. Then there's the type-A Wall Street stock trader who spends 16 hours a day screaming bloody murder until her blood pressure skyrockets and she has a stroke at the age of 42.

Golden handcuffs are alive and well, and many high-powered professionals are coming in at dawn and staying until bedtime, working 100-hour weeks in exchange for big, fat paychecks. Other, less privileged workers slave away just as hard, minus the fancy payout. Exceptionally long hours and unusually demanding workloads face physicians, investment bankers, business consultants, truckers, pilots, attorneys, and countless others.

Job stressors vary, but the stress affects the body in similar ways. There's the stress caused by interpersonal conflict, which may be experienced by lawyers, debt collectors, customer-service representatives, or anyone who is bullied by co-workers, supervisors, or customers. There's the stress experienced by people in high-stakes careers, such as doctors, nurses, firefighters, soldiers, air traffic controllers, commercial airline pilots, and criminal attorneys, where one wrong move can ruin someone's life.

There's the stress of jobs that expect you to sell your soul or sacrifice your integrity, like the advertising executive expected to spearhead a campaign for an unhealthy product, the white-collar insider command-ed to keep quiet about fraudulent activities the company might be en-gaging in, the soldier ordered to carry out an on operation he doesn't believe is ethical, and the politician who sacrifices her own values in order to get a law passed.

There's also the stress of feeling powerless or lacking control in the workplace, which might be experienced by the nurse who knows the doctor has ordered the wrong treatment but must follow orders anyway, or by the person low on the corporate ladder who has big ideas but doesn't think his little voice matters.

Other types of work stress fall under the heading of organizational constraints—tedious, frustrating hurdles that get in the way of getting the job done well, such as meddling co-workers, limited access to neces-sary information, or lacking the authority to do what needs to be done in order to successfully complete a task.

There's the stress of role confusion, which comes about when you don't understand what is expected of you or whether you're meeting expectations. There's also the stress of conflicting messages, when dif-ferent members of a work environment deliver countering instructions that leave you scratching your head.

While the mind interprets all these stressors as different, the lizard brain perceives the same thing in each case—*threat*. The physiological stress response flips on. Regardless of what causes the stress, the body manifests a physiological response similar to what happens when a per-son suffers from chronic loneliness. Because the mind communicates with the body via hormones, the physiological response is the same, whether you're listening to your boss rant at you, trying to calm down an angry client, or putting out a fire in a burning building.

So next time you choose to work overtime, your boss screams at you, or you're put in a work situation that leaves you feeling power-less, keep in mind that you might be taking years off your life by tax-ing your heart, wearing out your blood vessels, irritating your digestive tract, exhausting your adrenal glands, weakening your immune system, and stressing your pancreas.

Is it really worth it? It's easy to rationalize enduring stressful situations when you're working your way up the corporate ladder, struggling to keep your job in a lagging economy, or worrying about how you'll pay the rent if you don't make those sales. But are you really willing to withdraw years from your life account to make more money, attract more clients, or impress your boss?

Consider, instead, making an investment in your health for years to come by setting boundaries and implementing self-care at work. In Chapter 8, we'll talk about ways to protect your body from job stress, and in Part Three of the book, we'll discuss how to ensure that your work is aligned with your highest truth in order to optimize your health. Until we get there, suffice it to say that work stress is not benign. In order to live a vital, long life, it's important to find ways to feel peaceful and relaxed at work.

Typical Symptoms of Work Stress

When exposed to stress at work, the body whispers before it begins to yell. Before you collapse of a heart attack, keel over from a stroke, or wind up with cancer, you're likely to experience milder physical symptoms, such as backache, headache, eye strain, insomnia, fatigue, dizziness, appetite disturbances, and gastrointestinal distress.

Consider the following symptoms warning signs of more serious diseases in the making.

Backaches

Several studies have shown that backaches, such as those related to arthritis and fibromyalgia, increase in response to daily stressors such as work.[10] The relationship between work stress and backaches (as well as other types of musculoskeletal pain) is believed to occur because repetitive stress and activation of the HPA axis depletes cortisol and raises prolactin levels, thereby increasing the body's sensitivity to pain by suppressing the immune system and increasing inflammation.[11]

Headaches

As anyone who has ever pulled an all-nighter and suffered a migraine can attest, work stress can also cause headaches, most likely because pain-signaling pathways in the brain become hypersensitized in times of stress. Once the brain is overly sensitized to painful stimuli, even the slightest twinge may excite nerves in the brain, causing pain and muscle tension.[12]

Eye Strain

Occupational stress can also lead to eye strain, which includes itchy, heavy, or sore eyes as well as blurred or double vision, believed to be caused by inflammation and increased responsiveness to pain stimuli in and around the eyes. Certain workplace tasks, such as computer use, can also increase eye muscle fatigue.[13]

Insomnia

Notorious for keeping us up at night, work stress accounts for more lost sleep than any other cause.[14] A Swedish study showed that 10 to 40 percent of the working-age population reported work-related insomnia.[15] Scientists theorize that higher levels of ACTH and cortisol triggered by the stress response reduce surges of nighttime melatonin levels, which we need for restful sleep.[16]

Fatigue

Obviously, if your job is affecting your sleep, you're likely to feel fatigued, but other physiological factors may also make you feel fatigued when you're stressed at work, even if you're sleeping well. Although its mechanism is poorly understood, fatigue is one of the most common symptoms people experience when they're stressed by work. Work stress also increases the risk of chronic fatigue syndrome.[17] Theories link work-related fatigue to depleted cortisol levels, as well as to a genetic predisposition to stress-mediated fatigue.[18] What is clear is that individuals respond to the chemical alterations caused by stress in unique ways, so some people are more likely to feel fatigue when they experience work stress than others.[19]

Dizziness

As if some jobs aren't dizzying enough, workplace stress makes some people experience dizziness, believed to be related to changes in heart rate, blood pressure, and respiratory rate caused by stimulation of the sympathetic nervous system.[20] Alterations in these vital signs, particularly elevations in respiratory rate, can lead to hyperventilation, which alters the acid/base balance of the body, disrupting the nervous system's responses to balance and coordination via the cerebellum and the eighth cranial nerve.[21]

Appetite Disturbances

Depending on your unique physiology, work stress can either increase or decrease appetite, leading to weight loss or weight gain, although the most common response to work stress is decreased appetite.[22] Twenty-one percent of study respondents reported a significant loss of appetite following a stressful event.[23] Emotional stressors can trigger the brain to release ACTH and melanocyte-stimulating hormone (MSH), which can lead to loss of appetite and subsequent weight loss.[24]

Paradoxically, stimulation of the sympathetic nervous system may also cause the stomach to release the amino acid ghrelin, which makes you feel hungry and can lead to weight gain.[25] While these mechanisms come into play at the time of stress initiation, chronic work stress also affects appetite via stress-induced cortisol production. When cortisol levels are high, body fat tends to increase, and when cortisol levels are exhausted, release of the signaling peptide leptin decreases appetite.

Gastrointestinal Distress

Work stress commonly leads to gastrointestinal disorders such as nausea, heartburn, abdominal cramps, diarrhea, and irritable bowel syndrome, most likely meditated by the increased amounts of ACTH generated during the stress response. In response to ACTH, gastric emptying is delayed, which can lead to stomachaches and abdominal cramping. Heartburn can worsen, not only because stomach acid levels increase, but because the stress response reduces the stomach's pain threshold, increasing the perception of pain in response to heartburn and predisposition to stomach ulcers.[26] The stress response also lowers the stomach's ability to expand, which stimulates contractions of muscles in the colon and can lead to diarrhea and other symptoms of irritable bowel syndrome, most likely related to overproduction of CRF.[27]

Work Stress and Life-Threatening Disease

While backaches, stomachaches, and insomnia might not strike you as serious health issues, they are early warning signs, resulting from the body's stress response. These symptoms may be similar to the symptoms lonely people experience. The average American experiences 50 brief stress-response episodes each day, and lonely people or those unduly stressed about work experience even more, requiring the body to devote energy to maintaining healthy homeostasis.

At first, the body keeps up. But over time, the body gets tired and things go wrong. Frequent elevations in blood pressure result in thickening and tearing of blood vessel walls. Excessive production of fatty acids and glucose causes plaques that lead to heart disease. Chronic muscle tension and inflammation leads to pain and musculoskeletal disorders. Overproduction of cortisol suppresses the immune system, predisposing the body to infection and cancer.[28]

Chronic stimulation of the stress response caused by job stress can lead to heart disease, thyroid disease, ulcers, autoimmune disease, obesity, diabetes, sexual dysfunction, depression, anorexia nervosa, Cushing's syndrome, chronic fatigue syndrome, inflammatory disease, and cancer.[29] One study even showed that those in a hostile work environment are more likely to die young.[30] Another study of 7,000 people demonstrated that, while being employed is generally better for your health than being unemployed, it's better to be unemployed than employed in a badly paid, demanding, unsupportive job where you have little power or control.[31]

So while you might enjoy the paycheck a stressful job delivers, keep in mind that you may be paying a price even greater than what they're paying you.

Financial Stress and Health

If you're in a stressful job and suspect your health is suffering as a consequence, you may think about cutting back your hours, quitting your job, or switching careers. But if you're one of those people, the boogeyman in your lizard brain is probably whispering evil nothings like "You can't afford to quit, you moron. How will you ever pay the bills?"

This is a very real concern for many people. Your body might decompensate when you're in a stressful work environment, but the fear of job loss can amplify these feelings further.

Usually, work stress and financial stress are linked. It's a catch-22, really, because financial stress can be just as harmful to your health as work stress or loneliness. Studies linking wealth and health are numerous. Gopal Singh at the Department of Health and Human Services, along with Mohammad Siahpush, a professor at the University of Nebraska Medical Center, developed an index to measure social and economic conditions, using census data on education, income, poverty, housing, and other factors. What they found by examining data from 1998 to 2000 was that the affluent live 4.5 years longer than the poor (79.2 years versus 74.7 years). And according to Singh, this longevity gap is widening over time.[32] The affluent are less likely to get almost every disease out there except for cancer, and when they do get cancer, they're much more likely to survive.[33] They are less likely to have accidents or wind up disabled, and their babies are twice as likely to survive as those born into poor families.[34]

Rich people even suffer less than poor people before they die. In one study, researchers interviewed the surviving family members of 2,604 men and women aged 70 or older who had a net worth of $70,000 or more when they died. They found that the individuals with the highest net worth were 33 percent less likely to have suffered from pain in the year before they died. They were also less likely to have experienced depression or shortness of breath. These differences persisted even after researchers took into account the subjects' age, sex, ethnicity, education, and preexisting medical conditions. Why is this so? Researchers postulated that those with greater financial resources may express their symptoms more assertively and demand better care. They may also have greater access to services that health insurance might not cover.[35]

Of course, these disparities pose one of those chicken/egg conundrums. Are rich people able to earn more money because they're healthier? Are poor people financially disadvantaged because they're sick? Or do the wealthy just have access to better preventive health and exotic treatments because they can afford to pay for them?

You might argue that access to premium health care explains the divide, but studies show this is not the case. When offered the same health-insurance benefits, people higher up in a company's pecking order are healthier than those lower down.[36] Some health officials believe it's because social inequality itself is the killer. People of lower socioeconomic status may feel like they have less control over their lives and worry more about their basic needs, which activates the body's stress response.

You might be stressed because you just declared bankruptcy, your stocks went down, you got demoted, you're unemployed, or you can't afford to get food on the table. But even if none of these things are true, you could still be stressed at the very *idea* of them. The body can't differentiate between perceived financial stress (fear that you'll wind up flat broke) and real financial stress (you *really are* flat broke). Either way, the stress response becomes chronically activated, and this can translate into disease.

But it doesn't have to be this way. While you may not be able to change your financial status overnight, you can change how your mind responds to money worries.

Happy Workers Are Healthy Workers

Unsurprisingly, work environments that avoid shaming employees, encourage creativity, allow flexibility, and foster positive interoffice relationships have also been linked to better employee health. Those with effective employee wellness programs that are linked to financial incentives, such as Safeway, get bonus points for improving health outcomes in their workers.[37] But it's not just about making sure the workplace avoids shame and chooses healthy food for the cafeteria. There's also evidence that, while work stress can literally kill you, doing work you love just might save your life.[38]

Finding your professional bliss can be medicine for the mind, and the body responds with better health and more happiness. Happiness researcher Sonja Lyubomirsky, author of *The How of Happiness,* asserts that people who strive for something significant personally and professionally are happier than those who don't have strong dreams and aspirations. She says, "Find a happy person, and you will find a project."

Studies show that the process of working toward a goal and participating in challenging and stimulating work experiences is as important as actually achieving what it is you desire.[39] Committed pursuit of goals gives us a sense of mission, of pursuit, of being part of something bigger than ourselves, and studies show that this increases our sense of control over our lives, which is known to affect the health of the body.[40]

When your work involves pursuing goals that are personally resonant for you, it boosts your self-esteem as you start checking off the baby-step goals that get you closer to your big dream; it lifts you up and motivates you to keep on plugging away, doing what you love, even when the pursuit of these goals may require tedious tasks, risk-taking, and uncertainty. Pursuing goals also adds meaning and structure to our lives, keeping us on task, ensuring that the world will be a better place because we were in it. Striving to leave a legacy or pursue a calling increases happiness, which leaves the body flooded with health-inducing hormones that strengthen the immune system, relax the cardiovascular system, and deactivate the stress response.

Keep in mind that when I talk about "work," I'm talking about whatever you spend the majority of your day doing. For some, this is a paid position. Others might not get paid, but still work their butts off raising children, caring for ailing parents, or volunteering, and these jobs can be every bit as stressful as any profession, with equally negative effects on the body. They can also bring just as much meaning and purpose to your life, resulting in positive effects on the body.

The key is to remember that how our minds feel as we go about our day—how relaxed, happy, and fulfilled we are—gets translated into the physiology of the body. Way too many people subscribe to the TGIF mentality that leads them to dread Mondays, breathe a sigh of relief on hump day, and then drink way too much all weekend before putting their heads down and grinding away again at a job they don't enjoy. Or they quit a job they love to stay home with the kids, only to resent what they gave up, which leads to its own kind of stress.

However, when you feel free to be creative in your work, enjoy autonomy and respect, have clear goals and measures of achievement, are well supported by your co-workers, believe that your work is in line with your integrity, know that what you're doing helps other people, have a sense of mission and purpose, express your unique gifts in your work, get paid well, and spend enough time away from your work to pursue other activities, you're less likely to experience work stress and more likely to be optimally healthy.

Creativity and Health

It may seem peripheral to you to mention creativity as a factor in your health. Who ever heard of prescribing a hobby as preventive medicine or treatment for a disease? But scientific evidence shows that creative expression can elicit relaxation responses that counterbalance stress responses.

Sadly, being creative gets a bad rap in our society. From the time we're children, we are indoctrinated into thinking that science, math, and business are more valuable than art, music, theater, and writing. What our society seems to have forgotten is that being creative is not only fun; it's good for your health. Keep in mind that when I talk about expressing yourself creatively, I use a very loose definition of the word "creativity." I'm not limiting creativity to the arts. In some cases, your form of creative expression might be painting, dancing, playing an instrument, or writing poetry. But you may also express your creativity by scrapbooking, flower arranging, photography, gardening, interior decorating, blogging, knitting, hula-hoop dancing, singing in the shower, or brainstorming business ideas. You might express yourself by writing the perfect e-mail, developing a curriculum for Sunday school, cooking a gourmet meal, crafting music playlists on your iPod, salsa dancing, or generating ideas for new products at work. You might create workshops, design jewelry, or bake the perfect cupcake.

Whatever you do, flexing your creative muscles is as important to overall health and happiness as is flexing your biceps. The link between creativity and health has been well established, so anything that allows you to be more creative in your life benefits the physiology of your body and mind.[41] Creative expression releases endorphins and other feel-good neurotransmitters, reduces depression and anxiety, improves your immune function, relieves physical pain, and activates the parasympathetic nervous system, thereby lowering your heart rate, decreasing your blood pressure, slowing down your breathing, and lowering cortisol.

Health benefits of creative expression include improved sleep, better overall health, fewer doctor visits, less use of medication, and fewer vision problems. Creativity decreases symptoms of distress and improves quality of life for women with cancer; it strengthens positive feelings, alleviates distress, and helps clarify existential and spiritual issues; it lowers the risk of Alzheimer's disease, reduces anxiety, and improves mood, social functioning, and self-esteem.[42]

When we unleash the creative process, we tap into subconscious processes that help us heal—and thrive. Expressing yourself creatively exercises the right side of your brain, and doing so not only affects the body—it affects your emotional state, leading to greater happiness. And as we'll discuss in Chapter 7, it's a well-documented phenomenon that happy people are more likely to be healthy.

The health benefits of creativity are incredible—that's just how creative expression affects the individual! Creativity also affects your work life, your relationships, your sexuality, your spirituality, and your mental health. As art therapist Marti Hand teaches, expressing yourself creatively also promotes social peace by enhancing compassion, tolerance, kindness, harmony, expansion, growth, collaboration, respect, and healing. Even seemingly unrelated benefits may arise as the result of expressing yourself creatively, such as improved fertility.

While your creative life can be a potent source of physiological relaxation, it can also be a stressor if you're feeling creatively thwarted. One of my patients had been writing a novel in her head for years, but because she was so busy at work, her novel went unwritten. Every day, she felt stressed about the fact that she might die one day without ever writing her book. Creativity only heals you if you make the time to prioritize it. So don't forget about expressing yourself in your own way.

We all have a song within us longing to be sung as only we can sing it. As poet Mary Oliver writes, "Tell me, what is it you plan to do with your one wild and precious life?"

Rx for Job Stress

If you're feeling stressed about work or money, don't despair. You don't necessarily have to turn in your resignation letter or win the lottery in order to counteract the stress response. But you do have to have a serious heart-to-heart with yourself about how these issues might be affecting your health.

If you're committed to preventing disease or healing yourself from illness, be brave enough to tell yourself the truth. If you're concerned about how these stressors might be affecting your body, all is not lost. There's hope. You may be able to prevent disease or reverse illness by making positive changes aimed at bringing more relaxation into your body. If you're powerless to change your professional life, you still have the power to counteract at least a percentage of the negative effects of the stress response on your body with techniques clinically proven to activate the body's physiological relaxation response and improve your health. (I'll be discussing these health-inducing techniques in Chapter 8.)

But until then, know this: Stripping off the masks we wear in order to impress other people, appear more "professional," cover up our imperfections, and protect ourselves from getting hurt can work wonders when we're on a quest for optimal health. Being unapologetically who we are—not just at work, but at home, in the schoolyard, at church, wherever—soothes the mind, halts the stress response, induces the relaxation response, and heals the body. Authenticity, in work and in life, can be medicine for the body.

Chapter 7

HAPPINESS IS PREVENTIVE MEDICINE

"Happiness is not something ready made.

It comes from your own actions."

— HIS HOLINESS THE DALAI LAMA

It may seem obvious that happy, well-adjusted people are healthier. But when was the last time your doctor prescribed a program to learn optimism as a tool for preventing heart disease as effective as smoking cessation? When have you ever prescribed for yourself, as part of your preventive-medicine regimen, lifestyle modifications and practices scientifically proven to increase your happiness as a way of extending your life by seven and a half to ten years?

In modern medicine, emotional and mental health often take a back seat to biochemically rooted physical-health concerns. We tend to relegate emotional and mental health to the dark recesses of psychiatrists' offices, focusing instead on more physical preventive-health measures, such as a healthy diet, exercise, smoking cessation, and weight management. But the scientific data linking happiness and health is shocking enough that it just might convince you that treatments aimed at increasing happiness, along with happiness's twin sister, optimism, should take center stage when you're interested in preventing disease.

Multiple studies show that happiness and health are inextricably linked.[1] Sure, we all know that those who suffer from mental-health conditions such as depression, anxiety, or bipolar disorder are at increased risk of suicide, substance abuse, and other life-threatening conditions that directly affect the health of the body. But it might surprise you to realize you don't have to experience full-blown mental-health disorders that meet DSM-IV criteria for generalized anxiety disorder or major depression to have your mood affect your health. Simply feeling anxious, sad, angry, helpless, frustrated, or hopeless can trigger stress responses, and who doesn't feel that way at least some of the time?

Surveys of U.S. adults show that just over half (54 percent) rate themselves as "moderately mentally healthy" but not exactly flourishing.[2] Depression affects more than 21 million Americans annually and is the leading cause of disability in the United States for individuals ages 15 to 44. It is also the principal cause of 30,000 suicides in the U.S. each year.[3] Twenty-one percent of Americans will suffer from a mood disorder such as depression in their lifetime, 28 percent will suffer from an anxiety disorder, and one in five Americans takes psychiatric medications, mostly anti-depressants.[4]

Clearly, many people feel mentally unhealthy. But what exactly is happiness, and what does it have to do with the health of the body? Happiness researchers define happiness as "the overall appreciation of one's life-as-a-whole."[5] Essentially, it's a measure of how much you like the life you're living and how much enthusiasm you feel when you wake up every day.

The data is clear that unhappy people are much more likely to get physically sick. Depression, for example, increases your cancer risk, is a major risk factor for heart disease, and is linked to a variety of pain disorders.[6] Anxiety has been shown to increase cancer risk and increase carotid artery atherosclerosis, which predisposes to stroke.[7]

Happiness even affects life expectancy. People with higher levels of "subjective well-being" live up to ten years longer than those who don't.[8] Happiness also affects some health outcomes, including success rates of stem-cell transplantation, control of diabetes, rates of full-blown AIDS in HIV-positive patients, and recovery from stroke, heart surgery, and hip fracture.[9]

Studies show that positive psychological states, such as joy, happiness, and positive energy, as well as characteristics such as life satisfaction, hopefulness, optimism, and a sense of humor, result in lower mortality rates and extended longevity in both healthy and diseased populations.[10] In fact, happiness and related mental states reduce the risk or limit the severity of heart disease, lung disease, diabetes, hypertension, and colds. According to a Dutch study of elderly patients, upbeat mental states reduced an individual's risk of death by 50 percent over the study's nine-year duration.[11]

The Grant Study

The link between happiness and physical health became apparent during a landmark longitudinal study called the Grant Study, which followed upstanding, exceptionally gifted Harvard sophomores from three classes who were believed to be the pinnacle of physical fitness, mental health, and hope for the future. The goal was to watch how they lived their lives; pay attention to their health, happiness, relationships, and achievements; and hopefully learn how to predict, and thereby potentially control, why some people live happy, healthy, successful lives while others don't.

To choose just the right subjects for the Grant Study, Dr. Arlie Bock's team combed through medical records, academic records, and personal recommendations from the dean. The 268 Harvard students, mostly from the classes of 1942, '43, and '44, underwent evaluation by psychologists, social workers, physiologists, doctors, and pretty much everyone else Bock could assemble to record data about who these young men were as college sophomores.

Comprehensive medical examinations noted everything from organ function to the hanging length of the scrotum to brain activity as measured by electroencephalography. Social workers recorded bed-wetting habits, how the subjects received sex ed, and the family dynamics of their youth. The young men interpreted Rorschach inkblots, got their handwriting analyzed, and submitted to extensive psychiatric evaluation. All were deemed "normal," even "gifted."

The young men then graduated from college, but Bock, and those who took over for him over the years, studied them for the rest of their lives. The men were followed with extensive physical checkups, periodic interviews, and questionnaires, producing a veritable gold mine of information about what makes a person healthy, happy, and successful in life.

As the young men went off to fight in the wars that followed graduation from college, many of them endured the traumas that accompany combat. In spite of the challenges they faced, though, many of the men became quite successful. Four of them ran for U. S. Senate. One was a best-selling novelist, one became the editor of the *Washington Post,* one was a cabinet member, and one even became president. (It was later revealed that one of the Grant Study participants was John F. Kennedy.)

But as time went on, a trend began to emerge. By 1948, 20 of the young men displayed signs of severe psychiatric illness. By the time they turned 50, a third of them were mentally ill. Turns out that beneath the promising veneer of hopeful dean's-list sophomores lurked unexpected gremlins of the mind.

Quoted in an article in the *Atlantic,* Bock said, "They were normal when I picked them. It must have been the psychiatrists who screwed them up."[12]

Depression in these men turned out to be strongly linked to physical health. Of those diagnosed with depression by age 50, more than 70 percent had died or were chronically ill by 63. Those who reported being extremely satisfied with their lives had one-tenth the rate of severe illness or death compared to their unhappy counterparts. These findings held up after screening out other contributing factors, such as alcohol, tobacco, obesity, and ancestral longevity.[13]

Are Optimists Healthier than Pessimists?

Many years later, Martin Seligman, author of *Learned Optimism,* who studies optimism and its effects on life and health, was seeking a way to study whether optimists live longer than pessimists. For many years, he had been researching people's explanatory styles, how they explain unfortunate or fortunate events in their lives. As it turns out, the difference between optimists and pessimists lies in how permanent, pervasive, and personal they perceive good and bad events to be.

Because the pessimist views the bad event as permanent ("It'll always be this bad"), pervasive ("This is going to ruin everything"), and personal ("It's all my fault"), hopelessness ensues. When you make permanent, pervasive, and personal explanations for bad events that inevitably happen to everyone, you pave the way for chronic unhappiness and, ultimately, illness. Pessimists also believe that bad events are the result of their own failure. Good events, on the other hand, they believe to be temporary, specific, and outside of their control. Optimists, on the other hand, are a whole different breed. Optimists perceive bad events to be temporary, specific, and external, while they believe good events are permanent, pervasive, and the result of their own internal awesomeness.

Seligman and his colleagues sought out the Grant Study data to see if they could identify any correlations between explanatory style and disease risk. First, they had to determine whether optimism and pessimism are stable across a lifetime. Is it "once an optimist, always an optimist"? Or do people change?

What they found is that while optimism may change over time, the way people explain bad events tends to remain fixed throughout their lives. But that doesn't mean you can't convert. I'll discuss what you can do to become more optimistic and enjoy the health benefits that accompany optimism at the end of this chapter.

Once they realized that explanatory styles related to bad events tend to stay stable over time, Seligman and his partner, Chris Peterson, took a crack at the Grant Study data. What they found was that by the age of 45, the Grant Study pessimists were already less healthy than the optimists. The pessimistic men had started to get sick younger and more severely than the optimistic men. And by the age of 60, pessimists were significantly sicker.[14]

Turns out optimistic patients recover better from coronary bypass surgery, enjoy healthier immune systems, and live longer. They fare better when suffering from conditions such as cancer, heart disease, and kidney failure.[15] Optimists also live longer than pessimists. People with a positive outlook are 45 percent less likely to die within a specified period of time from all causes than negative thinkers (and 77 percent less likely to die from heart disease).[16] A positive attitude also affects our ability to ward off infection. In one study, healthy volunteers were interviewed about attitudes and then exposed to common cold and influenza viruses. Those with sunny dispositions were more resilient than those without.[17]

Other studies examining optimism versus pessimism followed. Harvard psychologist Laura Kubzansky, who studies optimism, tracked 1,300 men for ten years and found that heart-disease rates among optimists were half the rates in pessimists. The difference between the two groups was as dramatic as that seen between smokers and nonsmokers.[18]

As it turns out, pessimists are more susceptible to depression, more likely to experience barriers to professional success, less likely to experience pleasure, more likely to endure challenges in their relationships, and more likely to get sick.[19] Studies show that optimists catch fewer infectious diseases than pessimists, have stronger immune systems and lower blood pressures, live longer, and are less likely to suffer from cardiac disease.[20] In one study, pessimists had twice as many infectious diseases and twice as many doctor visits as optimists.[21]

A sense of positive well-being has been proven to protect your heart. Patients with high levels of "emotional vitality" were 19 percent less likely to develop coronary heart disease than those with lower levels.[22] And just to ice the cake, people with high self-esteem, who view themselves in a more positive light, have lower cardiovascular responses to stress, recover faster, and have lower baseline levels of the stress hormone cortisol.[23]

Hope Heals

When I was a medical student, I took care of a little boy named Joe, who had stage 4 cancer. Joe, who had never met his father, was in the middle of aggressive chemotherapy when he wrote a pleading letter telling his father how sick he was and begging him to fly to Florida so they could meet. Knowing the man's whereabouts, his mother promised to send the letter, and to Joe's delight, his father wrote back and promised to come see him in the hospital for the first time in his life.

As he waited for the visit from his father, Joe's cancer wasn't responding well to the treatment. His body was becoming progressively weaker. But Joe was an optimist. He believed he would recover from the cancer and have the rest of his long life to finally get to know his father, whom he had been fantasizing about for as long as he could remember.

At one point, Joe's organs began to shut down, and we were sure the end was near. His mother called his father to tell him to come quickly, and that night, Joe got word that his father had bought his plane ticket and would be arriving in a week. By the next day, Joe's condition had significantly improved, and he was up, walking around the ward, excitedly telling all the nurses about his father's impending visit.

The reunion was to happen on a Saturday. Joe spent the whole week making drawings for his father, writing stories, and practicing a song on his recorder to play for him. We were amazed at how sprightly Joe suddenly appeared, in anticipation of his father's visit.

Friday night, Joe couldn't sleep. My attending physician finally ordered a sleeping pill so Joe wouldn't be completely exhausted when his father arrived. Saturday morning, Joe begged us to let him out of the hospital so he could go to the airport and see his father the moment he walked off the plane. But Joe still needed his IV, and the doctor wouldn't let him go. Instead, Joe camped out on the front patio of the hospital in a wheelchair with his IV pole, where he waited with his mother and watched for the taxi that would bring his father to the hospital.

His father's plane was to arrive at 2:00. The airport wasn't far. He should have been there no later than 3:30. But 3:30 came and went. Joe waited. And waited. And waited. But his father never came. His mother called, but nobody picked up. Joe left messages, but nobody ever called back.

I was working that day, and I kept checking on Joe, who insisted his father's plane had been delayed or he was just stuck in traffic. But his mother had checked the flight. It had arrived right on schedule. Joe's mother tried to explain to him that his father wasn't very mature and didn't quite know how to be a father. But Joe wasn't buying it. He was certain his father was coming. Nothing could shake his faith.

I was on call that night, worried about Joe but running around, taking care of new admissions to the pediatric ward, when finally, at 11 P.M., eight hours after his father was supposed to arrive, Joe's mom was able to convince him to return to his room. When I saw Joe's wheelchair rolling through the halls and leaned in to hug him, Joe started crying and told me his father had stood him up. The whole ward—me, the nurses, Joe's mom—got misty-eyed as we watched Joe's thin little body shake with sobs.

Sometime around midnight, Joe finally fell asleep.

About five hours later, when I was still in the emergency room, writing up another history and physical exam as I admitted a baby with meningitis, the overhead speaker blared "Ninety-nine, Doctor Heart," our secret code for a code blue. Someone was dying, and as the medical student on call it was my job to be there. When I called the operator to find out where the code was happening, she gave me the room number.

My own heart almost stopped when I realized it was Joe's room.

Although he had been doing well the night before, Joe stopped breathing and our resuscitation efforts failed. Joe's dad never came, even when Joe's mother reluctantly invited him to the funeral.

You might say that hope had been keeping Joe alive—that's how powerful the effect of optimism can be. But while his story of hope withdrawn has a sad ending, Maria's story of how hope heals has a happy one. Maria was eight when she was diagnosed with a form of leukemia for which her doctors recommended toxic doses of chemotherapy, followed by a bone-marrow transplant. However, a transplant match couldn't be found. So Maria's parents made the radical choice to conceive a baby, hoping that the sibling would be a match.

While Maria's mother was pregnant, Maria's doctors treated Maria with lower doses of chemotherapy, which they believed would keep the leukemia in check but not cure her. The goal was to keep her alive until the baby was born, when cord blood collected at the time of birth could be screened and, they hoped, used for transplantation.

Maria, who had always wanted a sibling, was overjoyed that her mother was pregnant. Although the chemotherapy weakened her, her spirits stayed high, and she told all the nurses that her cancer was going away so she could be a good big sister. Not wanting to remove hope or interfere with her optimism, the nurses nodded in agreement, even though the blood tests revealed that the cancer was still there.

Maria tolerated the chemotherapy well, and a few months later, to the surprise of her doctors, her blood counts started to improve beyond what they expected with the low doses of chemotherapy they were using.

When the baby was born, Maria was in the room, outfitted with gear meant to protect her frail, susceptible body from infection. When she rocked her new sister in her arms, those present at the delivery were deeply moved.

But the cord blood collected at the time of delivery was not a close enough match for Maria. Maria's parents were devastated, but Maria told them not to worry, that her cancer had gone away and she didn't need the bone marrow transplant anymore. Her oncologists shook their heads. That would be impossible, they said. The doses of chemotherapy she had received were insufficient to result in cure.

But it turned out Maria was right. During her next round of tests, no trace of her cancer could be found. Although some might argue that the low doses of chemotherapy cured her, I believe hope and optimism did.

Learned Helplessness and Illness

When you work in a hospital, you often hear inspiring stories of optimism linked to disease remission and pessimism associated with disease progression. Martin Seligman claims that what differentiates the pessimists from the optimists is something he calls "learned helplessness." When things don't go the way we hope, we all—optimists and pessimists alike—feel temporarily helpless. When your boyfriend breaks up with you, your boss hands you your pink slip, your wife dies, your child is kidnapped, or you get slapped with a cancer diagnosis, you get the proverbial wind knocked out of you, and you're likely to experience negative emotions like sadness, anger, worry, and fear.

When bad things happen, however, the difference between optimists and pessimists is that optimists start to recover right away. Something in them knows they'll always land butter side up, even when they're in the thick of it. Optimists might feel demoralized, even temporarily depressed, but they pick themselves up, brush themselves off, and get back to the business of living a happy life.

Pessimists, on the other hand, continue to feel helpless over an extended period of time, which often spirals downward into full-blown clinical depression. Studies show that when pessimists fail—in relationships, in business, in the achievement of personal goals—they feel helpless, since it feels like the negative experience will last forever, will ruin everything, and has come about as the result of internal personal failure. Over time, they learn helplessness that leaves them feeling in the dumps, often for a long, long time.[24] We've long known that negative thoughts and stressors can make us sick, and researchers suspect that negative belief affects the body by triggering the stress response, turning off the body's natural self-repair mechanisms and predisposing the body to disease.[25]

Immune Response and Helplessness

On a mission to further elucidate the mechanism of how helplessness might be linked to illness, Madelon Visintainer, a colleague of Seligman's, performed a study on three groups of rats. The first group was given a mild, escapable shock—one the rats could avoid once they learned how. The second group was given a mild, inescapable shock, which rendered them helpless. The third group was given no shock at all.

Before setting about shocking these poor rats, Visintainer implanted a few cancer cells on each rat's flank. The cancer was the kind that would invariably kill the rat if the rat's immune system failed to fend it off. Visintainers carefully controlled the number of cancer cells she implanted so she could expect that, under normal conditions, about half the rats would reject the tumor and live. The other half would succumb and die.

Everything externally was perfectly controlled—the rats' diet, how they were housed, the tumor burden. The only difference among the three groups of rats was their psychological experience. The rats experiencing escapable shocks quickly learned how to game the system, ultimately avoiding the shocks. The rats getting inescapable shocks, on the other hand, were learning helplessness. And the unshocked rats were just minding their own business, with neither the challenge of figuring something out nor the trauma of getting shocked.

As expected, within a month, 50 percent of the unshocked rats had died, while the other 50 percent of unshocked rats fought off the tumor. But curiously, the rats given escapable shocks, who learned how to master the system, rejected the tumor 70 percent of the time, giving them a survival advantage over the unshocked rats. The rats who couldn't escape the shocks, however, wound up listless and helpless, and only 27 percent rejected the tumor.[26] From these rats, we may conclude that our sense of control, ability to avoid victimhood, and feelings of hopefulness regarding our experiences, particularly the traumas we face, may affect whether we get sick or stay healthy.

Based on this data, researchers concluded that learned helplessness in rats who couldn't escape the shocks must have suppressed the immune response known to fight off cancer cells in tumors of this sort. Further study of these helpless rats found that, indeed, inescapable shocks weaken the immune system. The T-cells of the helpless rats no longer multiplied and got down to the business of fighting off cancer cells when they came across invading outsiders. Natural killer cells, also important in fighting off cancers and other foreign invaders, lost their natural killer abilities. These studies confirmed what researchers had suspected. Psychological states can directly affect the outcome of remission from some diseases, at least those that are immune-mediated, as many cancers are.[27]

This may explain why optimists are healthier than pessimists. Because of their healthier explanatory styles in the face of negative life events, optimists are more likely to learn healthy adaptations in response to life's shocks, making them immune to states of helplessness. Pessimists, on the other hand, feel like life's shocks are inescapable, and like the listless, helpless rats, they get depressed and their immune systems weaken. Over the course of a lifetime, fewer episodes of learned helplessness may keep the immune system stronger, reduce stress responses and their negative health outcomes, and reduce the likelihood of disease.

Control as an Antidote to Helplessness

If rats can fight off cancer by exerting more control over their surroundings, is there any proof that humans respond the same way? Curious as to whether learned helplessness could be counteracted by increasing feelings of control, choice, and personal responsibility, researchers working with residents of a nursing home designed a study to evaluate the physical health of residents in response to positive changes made in the facility.

They divided the home into two groups—the first floor and the second. All residents would be able to enjoy the new benefits the home was offering—omelets versus scrambled eggs, movie night on Wednesdays or Thursdays, plants to enjoy in their own rooms if they wanted them. But in order to take advantage of these opportunities, first-floor residents were given extra choice and extra responsibility: they had to choose which eggs they wanted, sign up for Wednesdays versus Thursdays, and water their own plants.

Second-floor residents, on the other hand, were given the same opportunities, but they were offered no choices or personal responsibilities. Their schedules were set, leaving them essentially powerless. Mondays, Wednesdays, and Fridays were omelet days. Tuesdays and Thursdays were scrambled-egg days. They were assigned a movie night without being given a choice. And they didn't have to pick out or water their own plants.

A year and a half later, researchers found that the first-floor residents, the ones with choice and personal responsibility, were more active, happier, and less likely to have died during the study period.[28] As it turns out, choice, personal responsibility, and the ability to feel useful are good for your health, most likely because you feel happier, and this leaves the body better able to repair itself.

Cheerfulness Predicts Longevity

We know that unhappy people are less likely to eat well, exercise, and enjoy healthy sleep patterns. But the health consequences of unhappiness aren't explained solely by whether or not unhappy people neglect to care for their bodies. In 1986, David Snowdon began another longitudinal study like the Grant Study, but this time, instead of studying Harvard sophomores, it studied Roman Catholic nuns.

Typically, studying what makes people live longer is fraught with bias. For example, we know that people from Utah live longer than people from Nevada. But why? Is it because the ascetic Mormon lifestyle is healthier than the rough-and-tumble boozing, gambling, and smoking culture of Las Vegas and Reno? Do the people of Utah eat more nourishing foods? Is the air in Utah cleaner? Are Utah residents less stressed?

Because these kinds of variables make longevity studies tough to interpret, it's helpful to study populations for whom many of these variables are controlled. This is where the nun study comes in handy.

The health habits of these nuns were otherwise fairly well controlled—they ate roughly the same bland diet, they didn't smoke or drink, they didn't get married, have babies, or contract sexually transmitted diseases, their social and economic class was similar, and they all had the same access to good medical care. This made it easier to draw conclusions about what leads to a longer life. You'd think that such a similar population might have similar life expectancies, yet with all the typical confounding variables controlled, there was still wide variation in how long the nuns lived and how healthy they were.

Why the disparity? Upon joining the convent, new nuns were asked to write the story of their life up until that point (the average age of those who wrote these autobiographies was 22). By the time the study began, many of these nuns were already senior citizens. The autobiographies they had written many years earlier were used to assess their happiness in young life. From there on, the nuns were followed for the rest of their lifetimes.

One such sister was Cecilia O'Payne, who became a novice at the School Sisters of Notre Dame in 1932. In her autobiography, she wrote, "God started my life off well by bestowing upon me grace of inestimable value . . . The past year which I have spent as a candidate studying at Notre Dame College has been a very happy one. Now I look forward with eager joy to receiving the Holy Habit of Our Lady and to a life of union with Love Divine."

By contrast, another nun taking the same vows, Marguerite Donnelly, wrote, "I was born on September 26, 1909, the eldest of seven children, five girls and two boys . . . My candidate year was spent in the Motherhouse, teaching chemistry and second-year Latin at Notre Dame Institute. With God's grace, I intend to do my best for our Order, for the spread of religion and for my personal sanctification."

Can you spot the difference between the two? Cecilia used effervescent words like "very happy" and "eager joy," while Marguerite's prose contained no such cheerfulness.

So what became of these young nuns? As reported in Martin Seligman's book *Authentic Happiness,* at 98 years old, Cecilia O'Payne was reportedly still alive and hadn't been sick a day in her life. Marguerite Donnelly, on the other hand, had a stroke at 59 and died soon afterward.[29]

When researchers investigated the life stories of the nuns, they found that 90 percent of the most cheerful nuns were still alive at age 84, compared to only 34 percent of the least cheerful. In fact, 54 percent of the most cheerful nuns were still alive and kicking it at age 94, compared to 11 percent of the least cheerful. In general, happy nuns were found to live seven and a half years longer than their unhappy counterparts.[30] Other studies show that happy people live up to ten years longer than unhappy people.[31] Clearly, happiness is preventive medicine, and at the end of this chapter, we'll discuss how you can increase your happiness to assist your body's healing process.

The Physiology of Mood

So what happens to the body when the mind is in a dark place? Emotional suffering might start in the mind, but it is ultimately an embodied experience. You don't just experience unhappiness in your mind. You feel it in your body, as suffering cascades through your body via the stress response. When something hurts emotionally, an alarm is sounded. The stress response is triggered, even though there is no immediate bodily threat—just anger, disappointment, frustration, pessimism, heartbreak, grief, and other upsetting emotions. In this next section, we'll discuss the physiology of how anxiety and depression negatively affect the body and how happiness can heal it.

Anxiety

The amygdala, an almond-shaped group of nuclei located in the limbic system, deep within the medial temporal lobes of the brain, is the boss when it comes to processing and storing memories of various emotions. In fact, the amygdala experiences emotions even before the conscious brain does. Repetitive triggering of the stress response makes the amygdala more reactive to apparent threats, which stimulates the stress response, thereby further triggering the amygdala, on and on and on in a vicious cycle. The amygdala serves to help form "implicit memories," traces of past experiences that lie beneath conscious recognition. As the amygdala becomes more sensitized, it increasingly tinges those implicit memories with heightened residues of fear, causing the brain to experience ongoing anxiety that no longer has anything to do with the circumstances at hand.

At the same time, the hippocampus, which is critical for developing "explicit memories"—clear, conscious records of what really happened—gets worn down by the body's stress response. Cortisol and other glucocorticoids weaken synapses in the brain and inhibit formation of new ones. When the hippocampus is weakened, it's much harder to produce new neurons and thus make new memories. As a result, the painful, fearful experiences the sensitized amygdala records get programmed into implicit memory, while the weakened hippocampus fails to record new explicit memories.

When this happens, you wind up with no real memory of what set you off to begin with but with a very clear sense that something bad—something *very bad*—is happening. This explains why those who experience trauma can wind up triggered by situations that stimulate the unconscious mind when the conscious mind has no clue what's going on. You wind up feeling unsafe and anxious, without having any clue why.

Depression

Depression also leads to repetitive activation of the stress response, which, in a cyclic fashion, then leads to depressed mood. With all that cortisol floating around as a result of the stress response, norepinephrine, which normally helps you feel alert and energized, gets depleted, leaving you feeling apathetic and distracted. Cortisol also lowers the production of dopamine, which is important for helping you experience pleasurable feelings.

The stress response also reduces serotonin, the most important neurotransmitter responsible for positive mood. When serotonin levels drop, norepinephrine levels drop even further, sending you into a downward spiral.

In addition to triggering the stress response, negative emotions also enhance the production of pro-inflammatory cytokines, leading to inflammation, which has been linked to certain cancers, Alzheimer's disease, arthritis, osteoporosis, and cardiovascular disease. Furthermore, negative feelings can contribute to delayed wound healing and infection.[32]

When negative moods like pessimism, helplessness, hopelessness, anxiety, and depression prevail, the stress response flips on and stays on, leading to gastrointestinal disorders, greater vulnerability to infections and cancer, heart disease, endocrine disorders, and more.[33] Happy people appear to have stronger immune systems, as demonstrated by the fact that happy people develop about 50 percent more antibodies in response to flu vaccines and mount stronger immune responses.[34]

When you're unhappy, on the other hand, your immune system weakens, a finding that was confirmed by one study of grieving widowers demonstrating that T-cell multiplication slowed down during the grieving process.[35] Differences in immunity were also seen in a study of optimistic versus pessimistic HIV-positive women.[36]

Happiness

While the neuroscience of unhappy mental states has been heavily studied, happiness is less well understood. However, the advent of functional MRI machines, along with electroencephalography, has made it easier to study the science of happiness. From examining study subjects who reportedly feel blissed out, researchers have concluded that happiness appears to be located in the left prefrontal cortex of the brain.

But what activates this part of the brain? And what can we do to get our left prefrontal cortexes more activated? Most likely, the answer has something to do with neurotransmitters like dopamine, oxytocin, endorphins, nitric oxide, and serotonin.

Researchers break down "happiness" into two types of pleasurable feelings—the anticipation of something positive and the sensory pleasure of actually experiencing it. For example, you might feel happy fantasizing about your upcoming beach vacation in Bali, planning how you'll spend the end-of-year bonus you'll get at work if you do a good job, or visualizing the thrill of finally kissing the object of your affection. But you might also feel happy basking in the warm sun with crystalline blue waters lapping around your body, slipping on the new cashmere sweater you just bought with your end-of-year bonus, and caressing the soft lips of your lover as your body awakens with pleasure.

When you feel happy because you're anticipating something exciting, your brain lights up in the area of the nucleus accumbens, the pleasure center of the brain. Activation of this part of the brain is most likely related to the neurotransmitter dopamine, which mediates the transfer of positive emotions between the left prefrontal cortex and the emotional centers in the nucleus accumbens. People with sensitive dopamine receptors tend to have better moods.

Dopamine may be the primary neurotransmitter associated with the kind of happiness you get when you're moving toward a goal and then achieve it, whereas other neurotransmitters may be responsible for other types of happiness, such as feelings of love or the sensations of physical pleasure. For example, oxytocin, the "cuddle hormone," which plays a role in pair bonding and is released when you fall in love or snuggle your child, may explain part of how happiness affects your health. Made in the hypothalamus and secreted by the pituitary gland, oxytocin reduces inflammation by decreasing cytokines. It also indirectly inhibits release of ACTH, thereby down-regulating the HPA axis that gets triggered during the stress response. Happy people have been found to have lower levels of cortisol, most likely because happy people feel less stress, fear, anger, and other emotions known to trigger the stress response.

Oxytocin also activates serotonin receptors, lifting mood, and inhibits the amygdala, from which the fear that can trigger the stress response arises.[37] Oxytocin also stimulates the release of endorphins, nature's morphine, which reduce pain and can lead to euphoric feelings such as the "runner's high" some get while exercising. Endorphins, which are released by the pituitary gland during exercise, love, and excitement, trigger dopamine release, which then stimulates the nucleus accumbens and leads to feelings of pleasure. Feelings of sensory pleasure also stimulate the release of nitric oxide, a potent vasodilator, which increases blood flow and is known to be important in protecting certain organs from ischemic damage, which can occur when an organ doesn't get enough blood flow.

Most likely, happiness also affects the immune system, as demonstrated by the tumor-laden rats subjected to escapable and inescapable shocks. Learned helplessness, experienced not just by rats but by pessimists, who tend to be unhappy, makes the immune system more passive, leaving you more susceptible to infection, cancer, and other immune-mediated diseases. Optimists, who tend to be happier, are less prone to learned helplessness, which, over the course of a lifetime, may keep the immune system scrappier. The effect of fewer stress responses on the body, as well as the long-term consequences of a strong immune system, may explain the longevity differences between happy and unhappy people.

Does Happiness Cure Disease?

While copious evidence supports happiness as preventive medicine, predicting longevity in healthy populations,[38] what is less clear is whether happiness can also help treat existing disease. The data is mixed. Some studies show markedly improved disease recovery rates in happy people.[39] One small study, for example, evaluated 34 women suffering from a second bout of cancer at the National Cancer Institute, where they underwent extensive physical and psychological evaluations that included analysis of optimism. Because survival after a second bout of breast cancer is rare, after about a year, most of the women began to die, but a few survived. Who lived longest? The ones who were happiest.[40]

But while some studies suggest that a cheerful attitude and fighting spirit improve survival in sick patients, the data suggests that a positive attitude, while it may prevent disease, isn't always enough to fight disease once it exists.[41] In fact, some argue that the idea of fighting serious illness with happiness is a preposterous illusion that merely leaves the patient feeling blamed.[42]

Why, then, might happiness prevent disease but often fail to treat it?

It's hard to say, but most likely it's because the beneficial effect of happiness has more to do with the cumulative physiological effects of happiness on the body than with the ability of a happy or optimistic mood alone to cure the body once things have gone south. For example, it's clear that feeling happy can reduce lifetime exposure to the stress response, limiting lifetime cardiovascular risk. But once the coronary arteries are already blocked with atherosclerosis, perhaps a positive mood alone just ain't gonna hack it.

Another explanation for the disparity in data is that disease mechanisms vary, and the mechanisms of self-repair in the body also vary. Happiness, for example, has been shown to improve immune function, while learned helplessness weakens it. But for diseases unrelated to immune function, mood may have less of an impact on disease outcome. Although a person's mental state, mood, and attitude can certainly improve quality of life, it's likely that happiness can only take you so far with certain diseases. But since the data is mixed and happiness has other benefits, what have you got to lose by taking steps to feel happier?

Rx for Pessimism

If you're a pessimist prone to unhappiness, don't despair. According to happiness researchers, things like optimism and happiness can be learned, and you can enjoy the physical and mental health benefits as a result. In *Learned Optimism*, Martin Seligman teaches an exercise he calls the ABCs—an acronym for Adversity, Belief, and Consequences. When we encounter adversity, we think about the adverse event, and our thoughts are quickly translated into beliefs, which become habitual if we're not mindful of them. These beliefs have consequences that can affect the way we feel and the actions we choose to take. By learning to modulate how we translate adversity into belief and how we act on those beliefs, you can convert your negative thoughts into hopeful ones.

For example, say someone zips into the parking space you were eyeing (Adversity). You get upset and think, *That driver stole my place. That was a rude and selfish thing to do* (Belief). You get angry, roll down your window, and shout at the other driver (Consequences).

Or your best friend hasn't returned your phone calls (Adversity). You explain this by thinking, *I'm always selfish and inconsiderate. No wonder* (Belief). You feel depressed all day (Consequences).

Seligman recommends keeping an ABC diary for a few days to assess how you respond to adverse events. To do this, you have to tap into your internal dialogue and identify the beliefs that arise in the face of adversity. (Remember that beliefs are thoughts, not feelings. Feelings are actually consequences of your thoughts.) Then record the consequences—how you felt or how you acted in response to the beliefs that arose out of the adverse event. After reviewing the beliefs that arise in the face of adversity, pessimists may notice how the beliefs that arise trigger negative emotional states or behaviors, whereas optimists may notice that their beliefs help them overcome adversity quickly.

Here's the kicker. If you naturally tend toward pessimism, you can learn to change the beliefs that arise in the face of adversity, and by changing these beliefs, you can change the consequences and improve your health. Once you are aware of your knee-jerk pessimistic beliefs, Seligman recommends two ways to deal with them: distracting yourself and thinking about something else or disputing them.

To distract yourself from a pessimistic belief, try what researchers call a "thought-stopping technique" meant to interrupt habitual thought patterns, such as slamming the palm of your hand against a wall and yelling "STOP!" You can also ring a loud bell, carry around a three-by-five card with the word STOP in large red letters, or wear a rubber band around your wrist and snap it hard to stop the ruminations. Combining such techniques with attention shifting can produce longer-lasting results. When you shout "STOP!" or snap the rubber band, consciously concentrate on something else.

If that doesn't cut it, schedule time later in the day to ruminate on your pessimistic beliefs. Tell yourself, "Stop. I'll think this over later." Or write your thoughts down. Doing so breaks the rumination cycle and lessens the strength of the negative thoughts.

Even more effective than distracting yourself from your negative ruminations is disputing them. To do this, you have to learn how to argue with yourself. Review your pessimistic belief, tap into the wisdom of your wiser, loving, compassionate self, and make a case to prove yourself wrong. For example, if your best friend doesn't return your calls and your first thought is, *She hates me because I'm a terrible friend,* dispute the thought. Argue that she might be busy, that someone else might not have relayed the messages you left on her machine, that she probably meant to call but got distracted, that really she loves you and you're a good friend. In other words, the problem isn't permanent, pervasive, and personal; it's temporary, specific, and external. Based on this new optimistic belief, you can choose new consequences and abort the downward spiral that pessimistic beliefs trigger.

The keys to successfully disputing your negative beliefs include trying to find evidence that your negative belief is false (if it is), considering alternative interpretations of the adverse event other than the pessimistic explanations you've imagined, determining what payoff you may be gaining from such a negative belief, and if the belief really is true, thinking through the implications of such a belief. Let's return to the best friend who hasn't called you back. After thinking of alternative explanations for why she didn't call, examine why your mind might race straight to negative assumptions. Perhaps you're getting something out of feeling like a neglected victim. Perhaps you cling to your righteous anger when she doesn't call you back, and your payoff is that you get to feel superior.

If the real reason she didn't call you back *is* that she hates you because you're a terrible friend, what can you learn from this belief? How can you use this belief to learn to be a better friend? You'll ultimately realize that, if this friendship isn't destined to last, you can probably learn something about yourself from the relationship, and chances are good that there's someone else out there just itching for the title of your new BFF.

In other words, try to talk yourself out of your negative belief, and if you can't, let yourself think things through to the worst possible scenario so you realize that, even if it's true, the implications probably aren't the end of the world.

Seligman also recommends distancing yourself from your pessimistic beliefs, realizing that they are just that—beliefs, not facts—and concluding your inner dialogue with an energizing thought, one that lifts you up rather than dragging you down.

Are you a pessimist ready to argue with yourself and get happier? Your body will thank you if you do.

Rx for Unhappiness

Becoming happier and healthier requires more than simply shifting from pessimistic to optimistic explanations for adverse events. This is good news, because, according to the research of Sonja Lyubomirsky, 40 percent of our happiness is easily within our control.

Yes, it's true that 50 percent of happiness is dictated by a predetermined genetic set point. Happiness is related to activity in the left prefrontal cortex of the brain, and some of us just naturally have more active left prefrontal cortexes. Studies of twins have shown us that we're all predisposed to have a certain type of temperament. Some of us are naturally sunny, while others are inherently melancholy. While we can't change the genetic part of our personal happiness equation, we can make changes to our overall happiness, and the secret to happiness is probably not what you think.

Although you may think changing your life circumstances will make your happier—when you finally meet "the one," get the perfect job, score the deal, hit the bestseller list, get pregnant, or whatever else your heart desires—the research suggests that life circumstances only account for 10 percent of our happiness. Whether we're healthy or unhealthy, privileged or poor, beautiful or homely, married or single, or facing some sort of life transition or trauma, does affect us—but not as much as you might think.

Why don't life circumstances account for more of our happiness? Because of a powerful force psychologists call "hedonistic adaptation." When you finally attain something you want—the object of your affection, more money, higher status, greater beauty, or some material possession—it makes you happier for a short while. But you quickly return to your set point. When good things happen, we get a happiness boost, but it isn't sustainable. For example, newlyweds feel happier, usually for about two years, and then they return to their happiness set point.[43]

But here's the really good news! Forty percent of our happiness is unrelated to our genetic happiness set point and not subject to hedonistic adaptation. Scientific studies show that influencing this 40 percent can be as easy as keeping a gratitude journal every night.[44]

As described in *Authentic Happiness*, Martin Seligman conducted a study and taught a single happiness-inducing strategy to a group of severely depressed individuals. Although these people were so abysmally depressed they could barely climb out of bed, they were instructed to do one simple task every day: go to a website and write down three good things that happened to them that day. Within 15 days, their depression improved from "severely depressed" to "mildly to moderately depressed." Ninety-four percent of them reported feeling better!

In *The How of Happiness*, Sonja Lyubomirsky shares her findings from a study examining happy people. What she found was that the happiest people were not the richest, most beautiful, or most successful. Instead, as it turns out, the golden ticket to happiness lies not so much in changing our natural tendencies or even our life circumstances but in adopting certain behaviors that have been scientifically proven to increase happiness. In her study, happy people shared similar traits. They devoted a lot of time to nurturing their relationships with family and friends, were comfortable expressing gratitude for what they had, were the first to lend a helping hand, practiced optimism when imagining their futures, savored life's pleasures and tried to live in the moment, exercised frequently, were deeply committed to lifelong goals and ambitions, and showed poise and strength when facing life's inevitable challenges.

She also found that you can be happier by avoiding overthinking, cutting yourself loose from ruminating thoughts, eliminating social comparisons, taking action to solve problems right when they arise, seeking meaning amid stress, loss or trauma, practicing forgiveness, engaging in activities that get you "in the flow," smiling more, and making efforts to take care of your body.

I believe that living in alignment with your truth is also vital to happiness, and studies confirm this. Steve Cole and his colleagues at UCLA investigated HIV-positive gay men to determine whether how "out" or "closeted" they were with their homosexuality affected their disease progression. Study participants were asked to rate themselves as "definitely in the closet," "in the closet most of the time," "half in and half out," "out most of the time," or "completely out of the closet."

Researchers then followed the course of their disease. What did they find? On all counts, HIV infection advanced more quickly in direct proportion to how "in the closet" the patients were. The more they lived in alignment with their truth, the healthier they were. And the results weren't subtle. Those who were mostly or all the way in the closet hit critically low CD4 counts 40 percent faster than those who were mostly or all the way out, and they died 21 percent faster.[45]

When you make efforts to increase your happiness, the health of the body tends to follow.

Chapter 8

HOW TO COUNTERACT THE STRESS RESPONSE

"Within each of us is a spark. Call it a divine spark if you will,

but it is there and can light the way to health. There are no

incurable diseases, only incurable people."

— BERNIE SIEGEL, M.D.

Although it's common knowledge now, as recently as the 1960s, it was heresy for a doctor to suggest that stress and disease were linked. In fact, nobody even linked diseases like hypertension to stress, even though the word *tension* is part of the diagnosis. Doctors knew that patients tended to run higher blood pressures when they visited the doctor's office—they called it "white coat hypertension." But somehow, nobody thought through the implications of the fact that visiting the doctor can be anxiety-provoking and that such stress resulted in elevations of blood pressure that dropped once the patients went back home and relaxed.

Curious about whether there could be a link between stress and high blood pressure, Harvard cardiologist Dr. Herbert Benson started discussing it with his colleagues, who mostly thought he was wacko for even sug-

gesting it. But Benson was dogged in his pursuit of the answers, and finding none, he started researching the topic himself. Inspired by the work
of B. F. Skinner and Neal Miller on biofeedback and its ability to teach
the body to control apparently involuntary physiologic phenomena, he
started rewarding monkeys for increasing and decreasing their own blood
pressures. He signaled success to them by flashing colored lights. Eventu-
ally, he was able to train the monkeys to control their own blood pressure by simply signaling them with the lights. The monkeys were able to
control their blood pressure with nothing more than brainpower alone.

The study, which was published in 1969, caught the attention of
practitioners of Transcendental Meditation, which had been recently
popularized by the Beatles, Mia Farrow, and other celebrities. These
practitioners, who had heard that Benson was studying monkeys, believed they were lowering their blood pressures when they meditated,
but nobody had ever tried to prove it. Already on shaky ground at Harvard for wandering into the territory of what ultimately would be called
"mind-body medicine," Benson originally refused to do the study. But
the meditation advocates were persistent.

He then heard about another researcher, Robert Keith Wallace, who
was studying Transcendental Meditation for his doctoral dissertation at
the University of California, Irvine. The two decided to put their curious
heads together and collaborate on a study. Once they compiled the data,
they were shocked. The data was incontrovertible. Striking physiologic
changes accompanied meditation—sharp drops in heart rate, respiratory rate, and metabolic rate. In the initial study, the blood pressures of
the study subjects didn't drop during meditation, but overall, the study
group that meditated had significantly lower baseline blood pressures
than those who didn't.

Benson named the physiological changes that meditating people
experienced "the relaxation response," a term I've used throughout this
book as the opposite of "the stress response." He argued that, like the
stress response triggered when a part of the hypothalamus is stimulated,
the relaxation response is triggered when a different part of the hypothalamus is stimulated, as a safeguard intended to counterbalance the
emergency alarm the body sometimes sounds.

Benson was so impressed by the benefits he witnessed when patients practiced this simple technique that he asked himself the question—if a 10- to 20-minute meditation practice could result in such profound health benefits, what would happen with those who practiced advanced meditation? Rumors of seemingly impossible feats of physiological manipulation were swirling around at the time. Researchers who studied meditating monks had demonstrated that they were able to reduce their metabolic rate by 20 percent, something usually achieved only after four or five hours of sleep. This demonstrated that it was possible to manipulate "involuntary" mechanisms in the body exclusively through activities of the mind.

When he first approached Tibetan monks, they had no interest in being studied. Then Benson befriended the Dalai Lama, who supported his research. All of a sudden, the monks paid attention. He witnessed the monks, dressed in nothing but loincloths, wrapping themselves in wet sheets in freezing temperatures at 15,000 feet in the Himalayas. But instead of shivering, dropping their body temperatures, and possibly dying, the monks visualized fires in their bellies, raising their body temperatures enough to dry the wet sheets.

Benson realized that the fertile breeding ground of the relaxation response might be harnessed to implant thoughts in the mind by visualizing an outcome you wish to achieve—such as raising your body temperature, lowering your blood pressure, fighting your cancer, or alleviating back pain. He went on to study processes like these throughout his extensive career as a researcher. Over the years, Benson studied thousands of patients and published scores of articles in scholarly medical journals. Through this research, he elicited a list of the conditions that respond to the relaxation response. There are likely others, but he clearly proved efficacy in treating angina pectoris, cardiac arrhythmias, allergic skin reactions, anxiety, mild to moderate depression, bronchial asthma, herpes simplex, cough, constipation, diabetes mellitus, duodenal ulcers, dizziness, fatigue, hypertension, infertility, insomnia, nausea and vomiting during pregnancy, nervousness, postoperative swelling, premenstrual syndrome, rheumatoid arthritis, side effects of cancer, side effects of AIDS, and all forms of pain—backaches, headaches, abdominal pain, muscle pain, joint aches, postoperative pain, neck, arm, and leg pain.

In his 1975 book *The Relaxation Response,* Benson announced that he had discovered a counterbalance to the fight-or-flight response Cannon had described decades earlier. Just as the body has a natural survival mechanism built in to help you run away from a wild animal, the body also has an inducible, physiologic state of quietude, which allows the body to repair damage done by the fight-or-flight response.

After his book hit the *New York Times* bestseller list, Benson got a lot of media attention and was admonished by his peers because "physicians at Harvard do not write popular books." His colleagues continued to critique him, claiming that the relaxation response was merely a placebo effect. Because patients believed it would lower their blood pressure, it did. In other words, it was belief that made the technique effective, not the actual technique.

Because, at the time, he had as much disdain for the placebo effect as his colleagues did, Benson worked diligently to prove that the relaxation response was a distinct physiological state. What he found was that the relaxation response worked more than a placebo comparison; however, even though his technique was more effective than a placebo, the placebo arm of the study still worked 50 to 90 percent of the time. Benson realized that the placebo effect was not something to be scoffed at but rather something to harness. He proposed renaming the placebo effect "remembered wellness" and suggested that it was a useful counterpart to the verifiable physiological state those eliciting the relaxation response could induce.

Benson's continued research found that regular elicitation of the relaxation response could prevent and compensate for the damaging effects of stress on the body, preventing disease and sometimes treating it. Benson wanted to know if the same response could be elicited in other activities besides meditation, so he kept up his research and found four essential components that could reliably elicit the relaxation response: 1) a quiet environment; 2) a mental device, such as a repeated phrase, word, sound, or prayer; 3) a passive, nonjudgmental attitude; and 4) a comfortable position.

Later, he discovered that only the mental device and passive attitude were necessary. A runner with a mantra and a passive attitude could be jogging down a busy street and elicit a relaxation response. The same was true for those doing yoga or qigong, walking, swimming, knitting, rowing, sitting, standing, or singing. As he continued a lifetime of research, Benson found that the majority of medical problems were either caused by or exacerbated by the chronic effects of the stress response on the body. Other studies showed that over 60 percent of doctor visits could be attributed to the stress response.[1]

Intuitively, we know this, and when we're stressed out, we crave relaxation. But too often, we go about it the wrong way, seeking out unhealthy forms of stress relief like alcohol, tobacco, and illegal drugs, which only exacerbate the problem. There are, however, healthy ways to elicit the relaxation response—such as meditation—that are the best medicine we can take for treatment of life's stresses.

To test the effectiveness of elicitation of the relaxation response on the body, Benson invented a way to teach patients how to elicit this response in a way that wasn't as woo-woo as Transcendental Meditation or as spiritual as prayer.

HOW TO ELICIT THE RELAXATION RESPONSE
(From Herbert Benson's *The Relaxation Response*)

1. Pick a focus word, short phrase, or prayer that is firmly rooted in your belief system, such as "one," "peace," "The Lord is my shepherd," "Hail Mary, full of grace," "Shalom," or "Om."

2. Sit quietly in a comfortable position.

3. Close your eyes.

4. Relax your muscles, progressing from your feet to your calves, thighs, abdomen, shoulders, head, and neck.

5. Breathe slowly and naturally, and as you do, say your focus word, sound, phrase, or prayer silently to yourself as you exhale.

6. Assume a passive attitude. Don't worry about how well you're doing. When other thoughts come to mind, simply say to yourself, "Oh, well," and gently return to your repetition.

7. Continue for 10 to 20 minutes.

8. Do not stand immediately. Continue sitting quietly for a minute or so, allowing other thoughts to return. Then open your eyes and sit for another minute before rising.

9. Practice the technique once or twice daily. Good times to do so are before breakfast and before dinner.[2]

This technique was found to be highly effective for eliciting the relaxation response and improving health. But in his latest book, *Timeless Healing: The Power and Biology of Belief*, Benson provides updated information on how to elicit the relaxation response. Essentially, this is all you need.

A SIMPLIFIED WAY TO ELICIT THE RELAXATION RESPONSE

• Repetition of a word, sound, phrase, prayer, or muscular activity.

• Passively disregarding everyday thoughts that inevitably come to mind and returning to your repetition.

This can be done while exercising, making art, cooking, shopping, driving . . . whatever.

Meditation

You don't have to follow Benson's prescription for eliciting the relaxation response. Other forms of meditation offer great health benefits, which have been well documented. All forms of meditation, to some degree, activate the parasympathetic nervous system, decrease stress-related cortisol, reduce respiration and heart rate, reduce the metabolic rate, increase blood flow in the brain, increase activity in the left prefrontal cortex (which is observed in happier people), strengthen the immune system, and lead to a state of relaxation.[3]

Meditation also reduces pain, work stress, anxiety, and depression, promotes cardiovascular health, improves cognitive function, lowers blood pressure, reduces alcohol abuse, improves longevity, promotes healthy weight, reduces tension headaches, relieves asthma, controls blood sugar in diabetic patients, alleviates PMS, reduces chronic pain, improves immune function, and raises quality of life.[4]

Lest you, like Benson's colleagues, suspect this might all be due to the placebo effect, take note that one study even studied sham meditation and found that it wasn't as effective in improving health variables as real meditation.[5] I know you've heard before that meditation is a good idea, but it's not just good for your mind, it's a critical technique for countering the effects of chronic stress in your life and in your body.

How to Meditate

If Benson's approach to inducing the relaxation response doesn't do it for you, there are many other ways to meditate. Dr. Deepak Chopra recommends the RPM (Rise, Pee, Meditate) approach to meditation, suggesting that those who can will be well served to meditate first thing upon arising. However, if you, like me, have young children, you may find it easier to meditate when the kids are napping or away at school. If you work outside the home, you may find it easier to meditate over your lunch break or just before bed.

Regardless of when you do it, it's crucial to make the time in your schedule to help your body relax, whether via meditation or other activities, such as the ones we'll discuss later in this chapter. If you're the overachieving type like me, used to multitasking and cramming a dozen productive activities into a day, I know meditation can feel like a supreme waste of time. But remember, meditation *is* productive. You're doing this for your health. It's as important for your body as going to the gym, preparing healthy meals, and getting enough sleep—if not more important—so I strongly suggest you apply discipline and prioritize the 20 minutes it takes to help the body relax.

If your monkey mind races from thought to thought the way mine does, you may find yourself resistant to meditation. You may also find yourself tempted to skip it because the quiet time brings up emotions you're trying to avoid, eliciting feelings like grief, sadness, or anger. Or you may just find it boring. Whatever your excuse, I encourage you to try it, not just for the health of your body but also for the other benefits meditation can bring to your life, such as a stronger spiritual connection, a deeper understanding of your authentic truth, and a greater connection to the wisdom of your intuition.

If you've never meditated before, start by creating a peaceful environment. I have two altars I've created at home, one in my bedroom and one in my home office, which I sit in front of to meditate. My altars showcase objects that are sacred to me, such as a stone carved with the words "Love Life," a wrought-iron heart fitted into an iron box that I found in Big Sur, a piece of rose quartz a friend gave me, a condor feather, a small statue a patient gave me, a painting a dear friend made, a framed photo, a cup of sand from a sacred site, and several candles. When I sit down to meditate, I light the candles, burn some incense, and take a moment to let my altar soothe me.

Some people have rooms exclusively dedicated to meditation. Even a small closet can be tricked out to become a special space designed to help your body relax and your soul connect. Meditating outside can also be lovely. Because I live on the California coast, I often meditate by the ocean on a rocky beach that is usually deserted or in Muir Woods, among the peaceful redwoods. If you have access to quiet spots in nature, try a beach, a riverfront, a meadow, or a forest free of distractions.

The challenge is finding a quiet place where you will be undisturbed, ideally a place that helps you relax. Turn off the TV, silence your phone, and play soothing music if you like. The point is to create an environment conducive to freeing your mind from its daily clutter and relaxing your body.

If you're new to meditation, start with just 5 minutes per day and aim to work up to 20. Set a timer so you don't have to check your watch, and if you can, sit on the floor and close your eyes. You don't have to sit in the lotus position unless you want to, but sitting on the floor helps you feel grounded, connects you to Mother Earth, and roots you into your body when you meditate. Feel free to use pillows, cushions, and other props that help you feel comfortable. Keep your back straight so you can breathe deeply with ease. If sitting on the floor is too uncomfortable, sit in a chair and place your feet firmly on the floor to develop a sense of grounding.

Once you find a comfortable position, close your eyes to minimize visual distractions and try focusing on your breath as you inhale and exhale. Meditation teacher Jack Kornfield suggests that if you notice yourself remembering, planning, or fantasizing, refrain from judging yourself, but do call it out. "Hello, remembering." "Hello, planning." "Hello, fantasizing." Then return to the present moment, focusing on your breath. The minute you notice your thoughts starting to wander, come back to your breath and try to empty your mind. If your mind continues to wander and your breath isn't enough to empty your mind, try counting your breaths or repeating a mantra to clear it.

To circumvent distracting images that may appear in your mind, you may also try scanning your body for any parts that don't feel relaxed and visualizing your breath going to those tense spots. Imagine your breath as golden light flowing to the tense places and filling them with relaxation. Relax your back, your shoulders, your belly, your facial muscles. If you have trouble finding your tension, try tensing and releasing each muscle, starting at your forehead and moving down your body all the way to your toes.

You can also try visualizing a grounding cord, coming out of your bottom like an electrical cord or tree roots, dropping through the floor, coursing through the soil and into the bedrock, and landing at the core of the earth, where you can plug in. Allow anything that no longer serves you to release down that grounding cord, into the earth's center, where it can get recycled. You can also visualize this grounding energy of the earth's core coursing up through the grounding cord and filling you with healing light.

You may also try visualizing yourself in a real or imagined place of relaxation. Allow your mind to experience the relaxing place in a multisensory way. See it, feel it, smell it, taste it, and hear the sounds. If you're battling an illness, you might add healing visualization to your meditation. In your mind's eye, see the part of your body affected by the illness returning to wholeness and health in as much detail as you can muster.

If you find it too challenging to still your mind in silence, try guided meditation. To download a guided meditation of my voice leading you through a healing meditation designed to elicit the relaxation response, visit MindOverMedicineBook.com. Or try Belleruth Naparstek's Health Journeys guided imagery CDs.

Most important, don't judge yourself as you learn to meditate. Criticizing yourself for meditating "badly" or beating yourself up because your monkey mind won't calm down will only stress you out, defeating the purpose of making attempts to help your body relax so it can repair itself. Remain compassionate with yourself, and pat yourself on the back for any progress you make. Can't make it more than ten breaths into your meditation? Give yourself a hug and try again the next day. Like anything, it just takes practice. As someone who resisted meditation for most of my life, I can attest to the fact that it really does get easier with regular practice, and the benefits are so worth the effort.

Other Ways to Elicit the Relaxation Response

It's not just meditation that shuts off the stress response and calms the body. As we've learned, creative expression, sexual release, being with people you love, spending time with your spiritual community, doing work that feeds your soul, and other relaxing activities such as laughter, playing with pets, journaling, prayer, napping, yoga, getting a massage, reading, singing, playing a musical instrument, gardening, cooking, tai chi, going for a walk, taking a hot bath, and enjoying nature may also activate your parasympathetic nervous system and allow the body to return to a state of rest so it can go about the business of self-repair.

This is vital for every single one of us, not just as treatment for illness but for prevention of it and extension of our lives. Nearly 75 percent of people surveyed said their stress levels were so high they felt unhealthy.[6] But the relaxation response can serve as a counterbalancing response.

Can't quit your stressful job? Not ready to leave your unhappy marriage? Haven't found the love of your life yet? Not interested in going to church? That's okay. I'm not suggesting you have to do everything I've covered in this book in order to be optimally healthy. But I am suggesting that if you're exposed to stressors you either can't change or aren't ready to change, you must prioritize activities that induce the relaxation response as a way to counterbalance the stresses in your life.

Back when I was seeing 40 patients a day in my very stressful job as an OB/GYN, I would spend 12 hours a day practicing medicine and then come home to my art studio, where I'd paint until bedtime. I always said, "Medicine is my hemorrhage, but art is my transfusion."

What I didn't understand was that I was naturally prescribing treatment for my stressful life. While my physician job triggered my stress responses all day long, my painting elicited relaxation responses. Although I wasn't ready to quit my job, and although I wasn't meditating, I was still giving my body medicine, calming my body into a state of rest and self-repair for up to 40 hours per week in my spare time, allowing myself to slip into a state of creative flow, during which hours passed without my awareness of the passage of time.

Parasympathetic nervous system activation is the chill-out state of the mind and body. If your sympathetic nervous system got shut off, you'd stay alive (though you'd likely get eaten by that lion). But if your parasympathetic nervous system gets disconnected, you die. So the stress response is a change from the steady state of the body. It's the parasympathetic nervous system that quiets the mind, relaxes the body, and fosters a sense of tranquility. As Rick Hanson writes in *Buddha's Brain,* "If your body had a fire department, it would be the parasympathetic nervous system."

When the relaxation response is induced, the parasympathetic nervous system is in the driver's seat. Only in this relaxed state can the body's natural self-repair mechanisms go about the business of repairing what gets out of whack in the body, the way the body is designed.

The relaxation response also improves mood. It's hard to feel anxious or depressed when the parasympathetic nervous system is in charge. The relaxation response may even alter how your genes are expressed, acting like a Band-Aid for the stressed-out body and reducing the cellular damage of chronic stress.[7]

How will you initiate relaxation responses in your body to make your body ripe for miracles?

Rx for Self-Healing

Now that I've pointed out how the stress responses that originate in your mind and damage your body function, you might be expecting me to dole out a specific prescription for exactly how you can alleviate loneliness, find love, enjoy better sex, reduce work stress, earn more, be more creative, feel happier, and relax the body. After all, I'm a doctor. We write prescriptions, right?

Although we all crave quick fixes and long to believe that some expert finally has the one secret solution to all our problems, the truth is that you'd probably be annoyed if I tried to write your prescription for you. Any efforts on my part to do so, even those based on cold, hard science, would likely come across as trite. Just picture it.

If you don't believe you can get well, switch out your negative beliefs for positive ones. If you're lonely, join a club, get on Match.com, and find the right spiritual community. If you're stressed at work, quit and find a better job. If you feel creatively thwarted, start creating. If you're broke, earn more. If you're a pessimist, become an optimist. If you're unhappy, get happier. If you feel stressed, relax.

Easy for me to say.

Whether you're trying to recover from a health condition or prevent disease until you die of old age, the process is the same. In Part Three of this book, I'm going to teach you the six steps to healing yourself so you can write your own prescription. (Don't worry! No medical-school education required.)

Remember, I'm not suggesting you ditch your doctor. You should take advantage of all modern medicine has to offer to complement your self-healing prescription. I wouldn't recommend skipping that surgery when you have appendicitis or not taking that antibiotic when you have a severe infection. While writing your prescription will certainly increase your body's ability to repair itself when something does go wrong, I'd never want you to risk your life by delaying treatment if you're suffering from a potentially life- or limb-threatening disease.

Having said that, I highly recommend this process as adjunctive treatment, alongside any medical treatment plan you may make with your health-care providers, in order to speed your recovery, ensure an optimal outcome, and make your body ripe for disease remission.

Keep in mind that what I'm about to teach you works best for disease prevention and chronic health issues—not emergencies. It's also a surefire way to boost your vitality, your happiness, and your life expectancy. Whether you're sick and have hopes of one day getting off your daily medication, you're technically "well" but not feeling like you're as vital as you could be, or you're jonesing to optimize your already good health, The Prescription you're about to write for yourself is guaranteed to change your life.

Beyond the scope of this book, but bearing mention for those looking to achieve optimal health, are holistic and preventive health tips your conventional doctor might not bring up. While the treatment plan you're about to create is primarily aimed at healing your mind, it's not enough to care solely for the mind if your goal is optimal health. You can shift your beliefs from negative to positive, alleviate loneliness, eliminate work and financial stress, and treat your depression and anxiety, but if you're still drinking, smoking, and eating highly processed microwavable dinners, that just ain't gonna cut it. Not only does your mind need the right nutrition for healthy brain activity, the endorphins of regular exercise, and the rest of a good night's sleep, your body also needs to be nourished and protected from the hazards of our environment.

When patients on a mission to heal themselves from a "chronic" or "incurable" illness seek my guidance, I always recommend adding green juice as a daily supplement, eating as many raw foods (go veggies!) as you can, limiting meat or at least choosing animal products wisely, eliminating processed foods, adding superfoods like chlorella, spirulina, seaweed, and wheatgrass to your diet, taking a good multivitamin, and eliminating or at least cutting back on white sugar, gluten, caffeine, alcohol, tobacco, and illegal drugs. Under guidance from my raw foods teacher Tricia Barrett, I personally do a 21-day raw foods/green juice detox cleanse once every three months as preventive medicine, and I recommend the same cleanse to anyone trying to heal from an illness. (For more juicy details about how to use food as medicine, visit Juice DietCleanse.com or read Kris Carr's *Crazy Sexy Diet*.)

I also recommend optimizing the biochemistry of the body by visiting a conscious, open-minded functional-medicine or integrative-medicine doctor familiar with balancing and optimizing the body's hormones and neurotransmitters and using natural substances to boost the immune system and foster the body's natural healing powers.

I believe, too, that the environment in which you live affects your health. Are you living a "green" life? Are you being exposed to harmful chemicals in plastics, pesticides, lead, toxic household chemicals, mold, or asbestos? The World Health Organization (WHO) reports that 24 percent of global disease is caused by environmental exposures that could be averted. They estimate that more than 33 percent of diseases in children under the age of five are caused by environmental exposures and posit that addressing environmental issues could save as many as four million lives a year in children alone, mostly in developing countries.[8]

Clearly, you can do everything "right" when it comes to nurturing your mind, but if your body is full of poison, either from your diet, what you drink, or your environment, a healthy mind just won't counteract the damage you're inflicting upon your body.

Others address these issues in more detail, but what I'll cover is a six-step process for how to listen to your body, diagnose the root of what might be causing or exacerbating your illness, and create a treatment plan for yourself aimed at reducing stress responses and eliciting relaxation responses so the body can be returned to its natural capacity for self-healing. Are you ready to write The Prescription for yourself?

PART THREE

WRITE THE PRESCRIPTION

Chapter 9

RADICAL SELF-CARE

"The body says what words cannot."

— MARTHA GRAHAM

For many years as a physician, I operated under a false assumption. I spent 12 years training to become a doctor, ostensibly so that I would know more about the bodies of my patients than they did. Doctors are body experts, right? I was trained that patients come to doctors because they are broken and, supposedly, we know how to "fix" them.

Growing up with a physician father, I thought only doctors cured sick people. I didn't believe they could cure themselves. As a medical student and resident, I believed it was my responsibility to diagnose what was wrong with a person's body and prescribe the right treatment. If they got better, I credited myself. If they didn't, I blamed myself.

As a practicing physician, I felt the weight of my job—to make the right assessments, settle on the right diagnoses, and deliver the proper treatments without ever making a mistake. Aside from hoping my patients would participate in lifestyle modifications like smoking cessation, exercise, and a better diet, I didn't expect much of them. I certainly didn't expect them to heal their own bodies. That's what I was there for.

It's only recently that I had a sneaking suspicion I might have it all wrong. After all, who knows the patient's body better than the patient? While doctors may better know the names of the arteries in the hand or the muscles in the leg, in some cases, especially those related to stress, the patient is actually the best diagnostician. Perhaps, instead of believing we doctors know what's best for the body, patients should be diagnosing the root causes of their illnesses and writing their own prescriptions for what needs to change in their lives.

As I mentioned briefly in Chapter 4, I invited some of my patients to write what I called The Prescription for themselves. If they needed antibiotics, I wrote the script. If they needed a mammogram, I ordered it. But once we dealt with the lab tests, drugs, and procedures a patient might need, I invited them to take their healing process a step further.

I didn't just leave them to fend for themselves while writing The Prescription. Many were excited about the idea of partnering in their own care, but some expressed reservations or felt scared. My patients wanted direction and support as they navigated the process of making The Diagnosis and writing The Prescription for themselves. And in this chapter, I'll guide you through the same process I use with them.

Certainly, as a doctor, I believe it's my job to order the appropriate diagnostic tests and educate patients about the treatment options available. Herbert Benson promotes the idea of what he calls the "three-legged stool" of healing. One leg of the stool is medication, one leg is surgery and other medical procedures, and the third leg is self-care. His vision is that, one day, modern medicine will value all three legs of the healing stool equally, encouraging patients to play a vital role in their own health care. He suggests that treatment with self-care, using exercises such as the relaxation response technique we discussed in Chapter 8, would solve 60 to 90 percent of the problems that bring people to doctors, leaving the other two legs of the stool to round out the health-care experience.

After what I've learned in the process of researching and writing this book, I'm going to go out on a limb here and take Benson's idea even a step further. I would argue that medications and surgeries shouldn't even be given two whole legs of the whole health stool; that self-care, or, as I call it, "radical self-care," should bear much more than one-third of the weight. In our current system, if it's addressed at all, self-care is afforded little more than a brief mention after the drugs have been prescribed and the surgeries have been discussed.

Also, the self-care that may be discussed by physicians often stops short of addressing the many issues that contribute to disease. While nutritious food is medicine, exercise is vital, tobacco, alcohol, and illegal drugs can be poison, and taking your vitamins fills your body with what it needs to repair itself, these forms of self-care are not enough to counterbalance the effects of repetitive triggering of the stress response.

If you're lonely, you're stuck in a toxic relationship, you're full of resentment for people who have hurt you, you're cheating on your partner, you're selling your soul at work, or you feel spiritually bankrupt, no amount of veggies, gym visits, 12-step programs, or vitamins is going to cut it. Radical self-care also involves things like setting boundaries, living in alignment with your truth, surrounding yourself with love and a sense of connection, and spending time doing what you love. You need radical self-care, not just in your health habits, but in the rest of your life.

It's time for a serious paradigm shift, with doctors playing the role of educators, helping patients optimize all that Western medicine has to offer, teaching them about nutrition, exercise, and other preventive health strategies while also addressing lifestyle issues that may contribute to health problems, such as loneliness, work stress, financial worries, and pessimism. It's also the responsibility of health-care providers to educate and encourage our patients to make lifestyle choices that improve health, such as meditation and other spiritual practices, creative expression, sex, and healthy social interactions. Once we do our best to diagnose, educate, and deliver any conventional medicine treatments the patients choose, perhaps we belong in the back seat, leaving the patient in the driver's seat, with the doctor serving more as a trusted consultant than as the boss of the body.

I'll dig deeper into how health-care providers and patients might work together to facilitate such a process, but before I do, let me take off my white coat so I can tell you my personal story, not as the physician, but as the patient.

How I Healed Myself

By the time I was 33 years old, I was stressed out, burned out, and living in a near constant state of fear, anxiety, and overwhelm. I was extremely unhappy in my job as a full-time partner in a busy obstetrics and gynecology practice, where I was expected to see 40 patients a day and work 36- or 72-hour shifts in the hospital, performing surgeries and delivering babies.

On top of my stressful job, I was also twice divorced, I had lost several people I loved to cancer, and I was feeling profoundly lonely and depressed. Basically, my stress responses were firing off all day long, and it should have come as no surprise that my body was breaking down. But, at the time, that never occurred to me.

By the time I was in my 20s, I had been diagnosed with multiple health conditions, including high blood pressure; cardiac arrhythmias; a painful sexual disorder called vulvar vestibulitis; severe, debilitating allergies; and precancerous changes on my cervix.

I was taking seven medications, getting weekly allergy shots, and had undergone surgery on my cervix. But in spite of all the drugs and procedures, my blood pressure was still out of control, my allergies were so bad I could barely leave the house, I couldn't have sex without feeling like I was getting stabbed with a knife, my heartbeat was skipping around like a Mexican jumping bean, and my cervix still showed precancerous changes, even after surgery.

In short, I was a hot mess on my way to an early heart attack, and my doctors didn't know what to do with me.

I wound up marrying Matt, the love of my life, and my health improved to some degree after falling in love. But I was still loading up on drugs every day, and my body was far from well.

Then January of 2006 rolled around, when the Perfect Storm I described in the introduction hit. I became a new mother, lost my dog, my brother wound up in liver failure as a rare side effect of a common antibiotic, and my father died of a brain tumor—all within two weeks. Talk about triggering your stress responses!

Just when I was coming up for air, Matt, who was the full-time caregiver for our newborn, cut two fingers all the way off with a table saw.

Although the surgeon was able to replant them, Matt was unable to care for our daughter, Siena, for months. All hell broke loose in our lives.

These back-to-back events tipped my life upside down like I was a house ripped from its foundation in a tornado. With my stress responses on overdrive, it's no surprise my body, as well as my mental state, began to downslide again. I was nearly paralyzed from the emotional and physical pain I experienced. I wound up feeling like I was squished from all sides, succumbing to pressures I couldn't control that pushed me deeper and deeper down into a dark place, like I was stuck in the narrows of a birth canal, barely able to breathe.

But there was a bright side. The traumas I experienced during what I came to call my Perfect Storm put a crack in the armor I had been wearing to fit in and get by. When that crack ripped through me, I came to discover a long-lost part of myself I now call my Inner Pilot Light.

We all have this part within us. Your Inner Pilot Light is the radiant, sparkly spirit of you—call it your Highest Self, your Christ Consciousness, your Buddha Nature, or your soul. It's that part of you that is a little piece of divinity fueling your life in human form. It's that 100 percent authentic, never extinguished, always-shining-though-sometimes-dimmed part that lights the way back to wholeness, happiness, and health.

When I was deep in those narrows, I found within myself a brightness, a wisdom, a sense of knowing, like a perpetual nightlight or a guiding star. As the pressures from all sides grew more intense, the light within me grew brighter. And in those depths, I experienced an awakening, a homecoming of sorts, as if I was the prodigal daughter, finally returning back to my body after all those years of being gone.

My body had been whispering to me for over a decade, but I had been ignoring the whispers until finally, in order to really get my attention, my body began to yell. Once I started listening to my body and my Inner Pilot Light, I started knowing things about myself I just hadn't realized before. I gained clarity about what might be making me sick, what needed to change in my relationships, how I needed to alter my work life, and many other transformations I knew were inevitable.

Facing the life changes I knew I needed to make, I was terrified. Examining the truth about my life was like standing on the edge of a neck-breaking cliff and staring down into the vast unknown. I had a newborn baby, a temporarily disabled and unemployed husband, a mortgage, graduate-school debt, and no backup plan.

But my current life was killing me. When the pain of staying put exceeds the fear of the unknown, you leap. You do what it takes, even if you're quivering with apprehension. I knew if I didn't heal my life, I'd die young. As a new mother devoted to my family, I had much to live for, and I wasn't willing to let my desire to cling to the illusion of safety and security keep me from making the changes I knew I'd have to make to save my own life.

Now, mind you, healing yourself is not for the faint of heart. I had to grab myself by the ovaries and make some scary-ass choices. When I reflect back, I'm proud of myself for being so brave, and I'm so grateful to Matt for jumping off the proverbial cliff with me, because we were both afraid. We risked everything to save my life. And thank God we did.

I wound up leaving my job, which required selling my house, liquidating my retirement account, and paying a hefty fee to cover my malpractice "tail" in case anyone ever sued me in the future. We moved from busy, crowded, chaotic San Diego to a small, sleepy town near the coast in Northern California, where I spent two years licking my wounds, writing, painting, bonding with my daughter, and healing myself.

During the time I later called my "waiting and becoming" years, I gained clarity on my life purpose, deepened my relationship with my husband and new daughter, reconnected in a rich way with a Divine presence, and expressed my creativity in numerous ways. I also spent a lot of time in nature, practiced yoga, hiked every day, and reconnected with old friends I had lost touch with.

After two years away from my medical practice, I started feeling the pull to once again be of service, to fulfill my role as a healer. But I was nervous about putting my improving health at risk again. Then I was offered a job in an integrative medicine practice in the San Francisco Bay area, which I was reluctant to accept because the last thing I wanted was to leave my haven in the country and move back to the big city.

But the lovely physician in charge of the integrative medicine practice offered me the world—as much time as I wanted with my patients, the opportunity to use the beautiful, healing space to lead workshops, an invitation to showcase my art, and free rein to create a sacred practice aligned with my healer heart. I lit up like a Christmas tree and jumped at the chance.

Matt and I found a quiet glen of houses right on the coast near the Golden Gate Bridge, where I could live far from civilization, right where the redwoods and mountains meet the ocean. I had found heaven, and it was only a 20-minute drive on scenic Highway 1 to my new job.

Living in Marin County led me further down my own healing path. I met with spiritual counselors, started drinking loads of green juice, explored my erotic self, and climbed the mountains daily, all while I simultaneously started blogging and discovering the tribe of people committed to radical self-care and healing the world—the people I had been looking for my whole life. Suddenly, I was no longer lonely. I knew my life's purpose. I loved my work. My home environment was medicine for me. I was in love. And I was happier than I had ever been in my life.

One by one, I got off almost all of my medications and my health conditions either completely resolved or drastically improved. Today, I take only half the dose of one of my medications, I'm off all of my allergy shots, my cervix has returned to normal without further surgery, my sexual disorder is gone, my cardiac arrhythmia has disappeared, and my blood pressure has normalized. As an added bonus, I released 20 pounds of unhappiness weight, lifted my mood from depressed to frequent bouts of bliss, gained loads of energy, fulfilled multiple childhood dreams, filled my life with love, and wound up with more financial abundance than I had when I was working full time in my old practice. (For all the nitty-gritty details of The Prescription I wrote for myself, see Appendix C.)

My doctors were shocked. With little help from them, I had healed myself from conditions all conventional medical treatments had previously failed to treat. One doctor told me I had just added 30 years to my life. (She also told me I looked ten years younger. I didn't believe her until I got carded that night when I ordered a glass of wine.)

How did I heal myself? Although I also made changes to my diet and exercise regimen, I primarily credit the healing of my mind. I believe yours has the power to heal you too.

Making the Body Ripe for Miracles

Although my story may sound suspicious to you, I want you to understand that this is not woo-woo metaphysics I'm talking about here. It's simple biochemistry. In my estimation, most of my health conditions were stress-related, so making life changes that alleviated the havoc of repetitive stress responses and replaced stress responses with relaxation responses altered the physiology of my body.

This was no easy task. In order to heal, I had to lead myself through the nausea-inducing, heartbreaking process of diagnosing the root causes of why my body was acting up. (Hint: it wasn't just pressure in my arteries, a virus in my cervix, or histamine released into my bloodstream.) Armed with the scary truth about how choices in my personal life were translating into disease, I prescribed for myself life changes meant to transform my body from one under constant attack by the stress response to one primarily resting in a state of physiological relaxation.

Merely knowing what needs to change isn't enough. The hardest part of the process is mustering up the guts to actually do what you know you need to do. When you're happy, relaxed, and free of stress, the body can accomplish amazing, even miraculous, feats of self-repair. And in this state of relaxation, errors of DNA get fixed, enzymes catalyze repair processes, immune cells can get busy chomping up infectious agents, free radicals bite the dust, and repair cells spring to the rescue. The body is a miracle waiting to happen, if only we optimize its ability to do what it's made to do naturally.

I now understand that this is how the body works. When aspects of our lives are unhealthy, stress responses are triggered, and the body starts to speak to us in whispers. If we listen to the whispers, tap into the truth of what the body is telling us, and make changes that reduce stress responses and elicit relaxation responses, we can prevent the whispers from escalating into full-blown diseases.

But when we ignore the whispers—or when we're so dissociated from our bodies that we don't even hear the whispers—the body begins to yell. What started as a headache becomes a stroke. What began as a vague tightening in your chest becomes a heart attack. What was just the sound of blood rushing in your ears becomes an aneurysm.

When are we going to start listening to the body's whispers *before* the body breaks down? I beg you to start listening. Is your body whispering to you, or has it already started yelling? Are you ready to embark upon a self-healing journey of your own?

You might be thinking, *Sure, Lissa can diagnose the real reason she's sick and write The Prescription for herself. She's a doctor!*

But I promise you, you have everything you need to do this for yourself. If you're ready and willing, I'm here to teach you how to do this at home.

If you've done what you can to optimize conventional medicine and you're still sick, you're wanting to eliminate side effects by trying to get off some of your medications, you're hoping to avoid a non-urgent surgery, you're trying to achieve a health goal such as weight loss, or you're otherwise motivated to heal your body and your life, hop on the healing train and let's chug this choo-choo through the process of getting your body in optimal shape to heal itself. All aboard!

The Whole Health Cairn

In order to help my patients determine what life factors might be contributing to their health conditions, I developed a diagnostic and treatment wellness model I call the "Whole Health Cairn" based on the findings of my research, which incorporates not just how the mind can heal or harm the body, but also physical and environmental health factors that contribute to whole health. (I debuted the Whole Health Cairn in a popular TEDx talk I gave in 2011 called "The Shocking Truth about Your Health.")

In my medical training, I had been introduced to several wellness models—pie charts and pyramids that talked about nutrition, exercise, social health, mental health, and so forth. Most of the models included the body as the foundation upon which everything else in life builds. But something had always struck me as off about these models. Not only did I question whether the body was the foundation upon which everything else builds; I also didn't resonate with being able to take out pieces of wellness, like you'd cut out a slice of pie. I envisioned something more intertwined, where all aspects of health were interrelated, and the body was the sum total of the balance of all aspects of a wholly healthy life.

The vision for a new wellness model first came to me while I was hiking on a coastal trail near my beloved Northern California home. As an artist, I've always loved cairns—those stacks of balanced stones you see adorning beaches and marking hiking trails and sacred landmarks. I love the Zen of them, but most important, the simultaneous strength and fragility of them. A well-built cairn can withstand the crashing of the waves upon it, yet if you move one stone too far out of balance, the whole thing topples. All stones depend upon the others for stability.

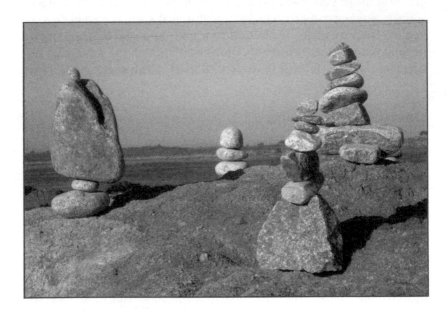

Like a cairn, the body is awe-inspiringly strong and resilient, and at the same time, fragile and easy to tip out of balance. If whole health is a stack of balanced stones, the body is the stone on top, the most precarious, the most likely to tumble if other stones shift. And as I learned on my own self-healing journey, the foundation stone, the one upon which everything else builds, is your Inner Pilot Light, that inner knowing, the healing wisdom of your body and soul that knows what's true for you and guides you, in your own unique way, back to better health.

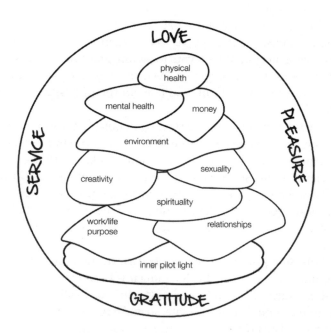

Atop the Inner Pilot Light lie all the other contributing factors that affect health—relationships, work/life purpose, creativity, spirituality, sexuality, money, mental health, and the environment. The very top of the Whole Health Cairn is where your body's physical health rests. The Whole Health Cairn is surrounded by the "Healing Bubble" of love, gratitude, service, and pleasure—the glue I believe holds everything in balance. Love and compassion—not just from loving family, friends, and health-care providers, but especially for yourself—are paramount when you're embarking upon a self-healing journey. Love opens your heart, trumps fear, and paves the way for healing in all aspects of your life.

Gratitude is also important. Without gratitude, you may focus only on what's lacking in your life, rather than what you appreciate. When that happens, this process can spiral you downward into overwhelm and despair, which only increase stress responses. You have to fill your cup and appreciate what you already have before you can face the truth about what isn't working and what might need to change. Gratitude keeps you optimistic, and as we've seen, evidence shows that optimism improves your health. When you focus on gratitude, positive things flow in more readily, making you even more grateful. As long as you keep your gratitude vessel full, you'll avoid the unhealthy plunge into dark places.

Service is another part of the Healing Bubble. Dedicating our lives to serving the world connects us to one another and reminds us to focus on something bigger than ourselves. Cami Walker, author of *29 Gifts,* treated her multiple sclerosis with a practice of giving one gift per day for 29 days, which sparked an entire movement. (Join others who are doing this at 29Gifts.org.) Committing your life to serving and healing others, even in small ways, can be big-time medicine for the body, mind, and soul.

And pleasure just makes the whole darn thing more fun, while also perking up the body with health-inducing hormones such as endorphins, dopamine, nitric oxide, and oxytocin. The healing process, while scary at times, should be pleasurable, so make sure you throw in a dollop of laughter, sensual pleasures, playfulness, and fun.

Each stone in the Whole Health Cairn is vital to the healing process, and the Healing Bubble contributes to the healthy hormonal milieu that provides just the right Petri dish for our minds to shift so our cells can heal. Keep in mind how important it is to keep your inner chatter positive during this process. If you let your inner critic (whom I call the "Gremlin") try to beat you into taking care of your body, it just doesn't work. If you're constantly telling yourself how fat, ugly, addicted, non-compliant, sick, lame, undisciplined, or worthless you are, this process simply won't work. You have to practice radical kindness with yourself, or you'll lose hope and fall into bad habits.

The only way to truly heal is to engage in radical self-care born of genuine love and compassion for yourself. Listening to the wise, caring voice of your Inner Pilot Light will help you do this. As you learn to send your Gremlin to time out, you'll find that you are your own best friend, and as you trust the knowing voice of your truth, your body will relax and your self-repair mechanisms will be able to kick in.

Most wellness models teach that the body is the foundation for everything in life, that without a healthy body, everything else suffers. But we've gotten it all backwards. The body isn't the foundation of your health. The body is the physical manifestation of the sum of your life experiences. When your life is out of alignment with your Inner Pilot Light and the stones of your Whole Health Cairn are out of balance, your mind gets stressed, and when your mind is under stress, your body suffers. The good news is that, if you're not optimally healthy, you can make changes that may profoundly affect your body's health.

As a Ph.D. student at the University of California, Berkeley, Kelly A. Turner became fascinated with those who experienced spontaneous remissions, and for her thesis she decided to travel the world interviewing two groups of people: patients who had experienced unexplainable remission from cancer and the non-allopathic healers who often helped this cohort of patients whom the medical establishment was otherwise unable to help.

Seventy interviews in places like the United States, China, Japan, New Zealand, Thailand, India, England, Ireland, Zambia, Zimbabwe, and Brazil were translated into more than 3,000 pages of transcripts, which she then analyzed to ferret out recurring themes. She identified more than 75 "treatments" for cancer, 6 of which were "very frequent" among all 70 subjects.

6 TREATMENTS THAT FOSTER SELF-HEALING
(compiled from the Ph.D. thesis of Kelly A. Turner[1])

- **Changing your diet.** The majority of interviewees credited diet change as a powerful tool for self-healing. Most recommended eating a diet consisting primarily of whole vegetables, fruits, grains, and beans, while eliminating meat, sugar, dairy, and refined grains.

- **Experiencing a deepening of spirituality.** Many of Turner's interviewees discussed feeling an internal sensation of divine, loving energy.

- **Feeling love/joy/happiness.** Others credited increasing love and happiness in their life with the ability to self-heal.

- **Releasing repressed emotions.** Many interviewees believed that it was healthy to release any negative emotions they had been harboring, such as fear, anger, and grief.

- **Taking herbs or vitamins.** Turner's interviewees took various forms of supplements, with the belief that they would help to detoxify their body and/or boost their immune systems.

- **Using intuition.** They talked about the importance of following their intuition with regard to treatment-related decisions.

These are the kinds of life changes that can make or break your fight against not just cancer, but any illness.

An Invitation to Heal

You don't have to wait until your body starts yelling with some life-threatening illness to make the same sorts of life changes. In the next chapter, I'm going to teach you a six-step process I use with patients, which has resulted in spontaneous remissions that can only be explained by the processes I've taught you up to this point in this book. This process is based on what I learned from the scientific data, and the results can be dramatic—not just with massive changes in health and happiness, but in whole-life transformation.

Before we move on to the six-step process, I should warn you that most of my patients cry. For many people, going through this process reveals blind spots they may have had for years, resulting in profound insights, psychological shadows from the past, grief in the present, and worry for the future. The Gremlins of self-doubt, self-criticism, and self-loathing can rear their ugly heads too. As I've said, healing yourself isn't for the faint of heart.

Why should you put yourself through what might be an uncomfortable process? Because you often have to break down to break through. This process offers you the opportunity for rebirth. As sung by the former Cat Stevens, Yusuf Islam, "To be what you must, you must give up what you are."

If you're fearless enough to face the truth about yourself, your life, and your illness, you'll have the opportunity to awaken to the bliss that comes with living in alignment with your Inner Pilot Light. And when you do, you relax your body, flip on your self-repair mechanisms, and make the body ripe for miracles. Remember, *anything is possible*.

But if you're not ready for this, don't worry. You've already learned a lot about what you might be able to change in your life to optimize your health, and if it's not the time to dig deeper, that is okay. Go in peace, and may you find optimal health in your own way.

If, however, you're ready to dig deeper, I want to encourage you to seek support from someone you trust, with whom you can share what might come up for you. Ideally this will be someone trained and experienced in the process of helping people navigate emotional issues when they arise, such as a therapist, counselor, psychiatrist, spiritual advisor, or life coach. As we discussed in Chapter 3, nobody should have to go through a healing journey alone, especially when we're talking about healing the mind.

Ideally this will be someone trained and experienced in the process of helping people navigate emotional issues when they arise, such as a therapist, counselor, psychiatrist, spiritual advisor, life coach, or graduate of the Whole Health Medicine Institute (WholeHealthMedicine Institute.com), where health-care providers are trained to help you navigate the six self-healing steps outlined in this book.

Keep in mind that terms like "healing yourself" and "self-healing" are misnomers, because they imply that you can do this all by yourself. What we should probably call it is "healing the body with the mind" or "mind-body healing," but that gets cumbersome. I've helped enough people through this process that I can guarantee you the process will be more effective and more pleasurable if you do this with someone.

Although I'd love to suggest that you enlist the help of your physician, unless your physician doesn't accept insurance and is able to devote a lot of time to you, I recommend finding someone with more than seven and a half minutes to devote to your healing process. The reality is that, as much as they might want to support your journey emotionally, most doctors simply don't have the time you'll need. You're probably better off finding someone who can spend a whole hour with you fairly frequently, someone like a therapist, health coach, or life coach. But if you discuss it with your physician and your doctor is up for it, more power to ya. And hallelujah! Nothing would make me happier.

Please trust me on this. If you decide to read the next chapter and do this process for yourself, find someone to be with you, someone who can allow your experience to be your experience without projecting their own fears, limiting beliefs, and life experiences onto you. Make sure you feel trust, lack of judgment, safety, and nurturing care, so that, if necessary, you can fall apart, knowing someone will be there to help put you back together again.

I also want to encourage you to be infinitely compassionate with yourself during this process. This is not an excuse to beat yourself up or shame yourself sick. It's an opportunity to illuminate what might lie at the root of your illness so you can make changes in your life aimed at optimizing your body's chances of feeling vital. Since I can't be with you, know that I am cosmically with you in spirit, and know that you are held in Divine Love, in the highest possible vibration, with an open heart and the faith that you can do this.

You have nothing to fear, my dear, and everything to gain. Everything you need already lies within you right in this moment. I'm just going to hold up a mirror so you can see what's right inside you. There within your answers lie.

——————————

Chapter 10

6 STEPS TO HEALING YOURSELF

"It's supposed to be a professional secret, but I'll tell you anyway.

We doctors do nothing. We only help and encourage the doctor within."

— ALBERT SCHWEITZER, M.D.

Before we get started, I want to make one final distinction. Throughout this book, I've used the words *healing* and *curing* interchangeably. When we talk about healing a fracture, we usually mean curing a fracture (the broken bone grows back together). In this instance, they mean the same thing. But the dictionary defines *heal* in two ways: "to effect cure" and "to become whole." From here on, when I use the word *heal* I'm referring to the second definition—the return to wholeness.

There's a difference between curing and this kind of healing. You can be cured without being healed, and you can be healed without being cured. In a perfect world, the process you're about to embark upon will both cure you and return you to wholeness. But I can't guarantee that you will be cured. What I can guarantee is that, if you embark upon this process with the support of the right people, you will wind up healed and whole, even if you're not cured.

When you're dealing with an illness, the process of being sick can be an opportunity for spiritual awakening, and when we wake up, we return to our natural state of wholeness. This state of wholeness puts the mind and body in an optimally relaxed state so the self-repair mechanisms of the body can best do their job.

If that's the case, why doesn't everyone wind up cured? Why does one person experience spontaneous remission and another doesn't? Some believe that all illness is the result of disordered thinking, that even if your conscious mind believes you can get well, you'll be sabotaged if your subconscious mind disagrees with you. Others believe that illness results from sins committed in a past life, which must be atoned for in this one—that it's karma. Still others cite divine destiny. And some believe that bad things just happen to good people and the "why" of it all is purely random.

I'm not here to discuss theology or spout off about things I don't fully understand, but I also don't want to skirt the issue altogether. So what's my answer to why some are cured when they heal their minds and others aren't? All I can say is this: when my patients have been brave, optimistic, and willing to do whatever it takes to heal, seemingly miraculous feats of physical self-repair have sometimes happened. The same thing can happen to you. So come on. You have everything to gain as you reclaim who you really are, align with your truth, and make your body ripe for miracles. Whether or not you cure your body, I guarantee your life will improve if you follow the steps I'm about to teach you. I believe in you, so please . . . come with me.

6 STEPS TO HEALING YOURSELF

STEP ONE: Believe You Can Heal Yourself

What the placebo and nocebo data taught us is that if you're plagued by negative, self-sabotaging beliefs about your health, either consciously or subconsciously, any attempt to heal yourself may be limited. What you believe manifests in the body. Most people believe certain illnesses are incurable, terminal, or chronic, but what if such beliefs are simply false?

For a long time, people believed that it was physiologically impossible for a human being to run a mile in less than four minutes. As long as everybody believed it to be true, nobody ever ran a sub-four-minute mile. Then something radical happened.

In 1954, Roger Bannister proved the sports physiologists wrong by running the mile in 3 minutes and 59 seconds for the first time in recorded history. Suddenly, the worldwide belief that running a sub-four-minute mile was physiologically impossible disappeared. Shortly thereafter, several other runners went on to run a mile in less than four minutes. In one famous race only 46 days later, Roger Bannister and John Landy both ran the mile in under four minutes, with Bannister winning the race.

Leading up to this time, athletes had been running faster and faster, but the four-minute mark seemed to erect a real physiological barrier nobody could overcome. It's as if the body simply couldn't cross over because the mind held this belief. But as soon as the belief was shattered by Bannister, the body was able to accomplish seemingly miraculous feats of athleticism.

Now, with the limiting belief that it was physiologically impossible shattered, virtually every athlete who competes in a world-class event has run the mile in under four minutes. Today's world-record time for the mile is 3:43:15, more than 15 seconds under 4 minutes.

What if believing that certain diseases cannot be cured is simply a limiting belief like the one that limited the athletes who longed to break the four-minute mile? What if you changed that self-sabotaging belief and allowed for the possibility that you, like the people whose medical miracles were reported in the Spontaneous Remission Project and the cancer patients Kelly Turner studied, might be free of what others might consider an incurable illness?

Just like the athletes who couldn't run the sub-four-minute mile—and then did—your beliefs may be limiting what your body can do. As long as you believe your disease is incurable, this will be a self-fulfilling prophecy. But what if simply changing your mind could alter your brain, while simultaneously altering your body's physiology?

Let me invite you to open your mind. Shift your beliefs. Make room for the "impossible." You just never know what miracles might happen.

Remember the meditating monks who could visualize a fire in their bellies and increase their body temperatures? You, too, can change your physiology with the power of your thoughts. It helps to start with meditation. Quieting your mind makes it more receptive to changing beliefs. Try using the relaxation response or other meditation techniques described in Chapter 8. While you're meditating and your mind and body are in a state of physiological rest and receptivity, try repeating positive affirmations to yourself. Create statements that affirm how you want your body to feel, such as "I am whole, healthy, and free of symptoms." Repeat these affirmations to yourself throughout the day.

You can also try visualizing your healthy body like a movie in your mind. Close your eyes, take a few deep breaths, and see your body cured of all illness in your mind's eye. Be as specific as you can in your visualization. Look up the anatomy and physiology of your illness if necessary so you know what the diseased organ looks like when healthy. See yourself disease-free and vital. Get sensory. Feel, see, smell, hear, even taste your new reality in as much detail as you can muster in your imagination. Detailed visualization and affirmations help the brain imprint the new belief into the subconscious mind.

It's also important to be the guardian of your brain. You may not realize the power of the messages you allow into your brain. Make a conscious effort to avoid negative thoughts about your health, such as *I'm going to get cancer because my mother did* or *I'm an unhealthy person.* Replace your conscious negative thoughts with positive affirmations. Also, in your mind, focus on what you want, not what you *don't* want. The subconscious mind doesn't process negation, so when you tell your mind, "I don't want to believe I'll be sick my whole life," it hears, "I do want to believe I'll be sick my whole life."

To go deeper into changing beliefs at the level of the subconscious mind, consider techniques such as hypnotherapy, Psych-K, Emotional Freedom Technique (EFT), and Neuro-Linguistic Programming (NLP). Hypnosis bypasses the conscious mind and digs straight into the subconscious mind, allowing beliefs to change more quickly. Psych-K synchronizes your right and left brain while you repeat positive affirmations and feel into the outcome you wish to achieve. EFT (also known as "tapping" therapy) has you tap your fingers along acupressure points while repeating positive affirmations. And NLP is based on the premise that how we choose our words reflects our inner, subconscious beliefs, and by changing our words, we can shift belief and heal problem areas in our lives. All are useful for shifting limiting, self-sabotaging beliefs and reprogramming the subconscious mind.

STEP TWO: Find the Right Support

As previously discussed, although your mind has the power to heal your body, you won't want to navigate this journey solo. Not only will you need a therapist, life coach, or someone else to guide you, you'll also want to optimize whatever potential cures physicians and modern medicine have to offer as an adjunct to healing your mind. When embarking on a healing journey, it takes a village. How do you find the right team of people to sit at your healing round table? Here are some tips.

Interview your team. Let them know when you make the appointment that you would like to schedule a consultation to make sure the fit is right. If the doctor, therapist, life coach, or other health-care provider won't submit to being interviewed, find someone who will. The right health-care providers will not be insulted by your request. But be prepared to pay out of pocket for such an interview. Your insurance may not cover it.

Find health-care providers who believe in you. The scientific data suggests that if your health-care provider believes you will get well, you're more likely to thrive. Feel free to ask your provider flat out, "Do you believe I can get better?" Pay close attention to the answer. If your doctor reads you negative statistics, insists that the outlook is not good, labels you as "incurable," and generally considers you a hopeless case, you might think about finding someone else. Keep in mind that as physicians, we are trained to be "realists" (a.k.a. "pessimists"). But don't be afraid to communicate your positive beliefs to your doctors. Offer your health-care providers copies of this book and ask if they're willing to partner with you. When invited to approach the treatment of an illness with optimism, many physicians will change their tune and appreciate the reminder that positive thinking does not equal false hope.

Seek health-care providers who truly care. It's time to bring the "care" back to health care. You are more than a room number or a body part. If your provider can't treat you like the whole, fabulous human being you are, keep looking and find someone who can. There are loads of talented, nurturing practitioners with remarkable skills, excellent bedside manners, and big, wide-open hearts just waiting for a wonderful patient like you.

Put your body in the hands of providers willing to collaborate. If your homeopath hates doctors, and your doctor thinks your Reiki master is a quack, it's going to be hard to get everyone on the same page. If you're assembling a team that includes healers outside the scope of conventional medicine, make sure your providers are willing and eager to communicate respectfully with each other so you don't wind up getting conflicting advice that not only confuses you, but can be downright dangerous.

Listen to the wisdom of your body. What does your gut say when you're with your health-care provider? Do you feel safe in her hands? Do you trust him? Do you think you'll get sound medical advice or do you get a weird vibe? Check in with how your body reacts. If you feel tight, clenched, nervous, cold, shivery, or closed off, your body may be telling you something. Look for feelings of openness, warmth, relaxation, and calmness in your body.

Make sure your health-care provider respects your intuition. If you question a treatment and express your opinion in a respectful manner and your intuition isn't respected, you might think twice about whether this is the best provider for you. As health-care providers, our job is to present you with your options, educate you about the risks and benefits, and make treatment recommendations, but ultimately, the choice is 100 percent yours. If your practitioner gets her panties in a wad because you don't choose to follow her recommendations, it's her problem, not yours. The right practitioner will welcome your feedback, understand that you know your body better than anybody else, and respect your wishes.

Be willing to sign a waiver. In today's litigious society, your practitioners or their malpractice-insurance carriers may require that you sign a waiver if you opt to decline the treatment they recommend but still wish to be a patient under their care. Don't take it personally. They're just covering their butts, and it doesn't mean that they don't support your autonomy.

Know that you deserve the best care possible. Don't go telling yourself stories about how you're not good enough/smart enough/ young enough/rich enough/[fill in the blank] enough to get this kind of stellar medical care. You may have to pay out of pocket to get it, since some forward-thinking doctors have opted out of the insurance system in order to offer premium health care and more time with patients. But what is more important than your health? Know that you are worth the best health care possible.

STEP THREE: Listen to Your Body and Intuition

Your Inner Pilot Light, the wise healer that lies within you, is your body's best friend and always knows exactly what your body needs. But many have unwittingly distanced themselves from the wisdom of their Inner Pilot Lights. Often, this is because we no longer reside in our own bodies. Instead of living embodied lives, heeding the wisdom of our intuition, and feeling all five senses in our own skin, we dissociate. Doctors know this better than anyone.

As a physician-in-training, I was expected to work almost constantly, so I wasn't free to sleep when I was tired, eat when I was hungry, pee when my bladder was full, quit operating when my shoulders got sore, or stay home and rest when I was sick. I had to soldier on, no matter what my body was telling me.

I was also too busy to listen to the quiet whispers of my intuitive knowing. Usually, I had to get whacked upside the head with the pro-verbial two-by-four. My body had to yell before I would notice that I had gotten off track in my life. As a defense against recurrent pain and dis-comfort, I learned to be a walking cerebrum, living an out-of-body expe-rience. While doctors, athletes, and soldiers may be extreme examples of how we learn to get out of our bodies so we don't experience physical or emotional pain, most of us experience some level of mind-body dis-sociation as an adaptation that later comes around to bite us. When we dissociate from the body, we don't hear the whispers the body delivers as warning signs intended to whip us into shape.

But you can change all that. If you're having trouble tapping into the healing wisdom of your Inner Pilot Light, try using your body as a brilliant entry point into your intuition about what will help your body heal. When you learn to listen to the wisdom your body is sharing with you, you will find all the answers you need in order to know how to navigate your self-healing journey. You'll also learn how to prevent fu-ture illness by noticing the whispers from your body before they become rebel yells. (See Appendix A for 8 Tips for How to Be in Your Body.)

Try these exercises intended to help you tap into the wisdom of your Inner Pilot Light as it communicates through your body.

Exercise: Let Your Body Be Your Guide

1. **Get quiet.** Spend a few moments sitting down, closing your eyes.

2. **Breathe deeply.** Notice your chest as it rises and falls. Feel the sensation of air hitting your nostrils.

3. **Notice any physical sensations you experience.** Do you feel pain? Tightness? Buzzing? Warmth? Cold? Openness? Constric-tion? Physical symptoms of an illness?

4. **Ask your body what it's trying to communicate to you.** Invite your Inner Pilot Light to answer. Listen to the wisdom of what comes up.

5. **Now open your eyes and let your physical symptom or illness write you a letter.** For example, if you have back pain, let your back pain write to you. (Dear You, Love, Your Back Pain.) If you have cancer, let your cancer pen the letter. (Dear You, Love, Your Cancer.)

6. **Write a response.** Once your physical symptom or illness has written to you, write back. (Dear Back Pain, Love, Me.)

7. **Let the back-and-forth dialogue ensue as long as you're learning from your body.** Take notice of what comes up in the letters. This is your Inner Pilot Light speaking. Listen up.

8. **Thank your body for its wisdom.** Promise to keep in touch more often.

Often, we choose to ignore the messages sent to us from our Inner Pilot Lights via the body, either because we're not listening or because we don't like what the messages have to say. Tapping into this body wisdom may command change, and we may not be fond of hearing those messages if we're not yet ready to change.

For example, a nagging cough may be your body's way of telling you it's time to quit smoking, but if you're not willing to quit, you'll likely distance yourself from your Inner Pilot Light. A lump in your neck may tell you it's time to go to the doctor, but if you're afraid of what you might hear, you may ignore it until the lump becomes so great that you lose your voice. Pain during sex may be your body's way of saying it no longer feels safe in your relationship and it's time to move on. Cancer or a heart attack may be telling you to *slow down.*

If you let them, physical symptoms can build a bridge between you and your Inner Pilot Light. When you learn to listen to the nuances of what your Inner Pilot Light is telling you, the body will no longer have to manifest these messages physically, and you may prevent physical symptoms or serious disease. But if you're not skilled at hearing this internal voice, your body can be your guide. Within your body lies the perfect compass that will guide you back home, if only you listen.

For more tips on tapping into the wisdom of your Inner Pilot Light, sign up for inspiring daily messages at InnerPilotLight.com.

STEP FOUR: Diagnose the Root Causes of Your Illness

If you have a health condition, your doctor may have already given you a diagnosis—angina, Crohn's disease, diabetes, breast cancer, whatever. As I've said before, if you're experiencing symptoms and haven't yet seen a doctor, please get to it—pronto. We've come a long way in the past century, and modern medicine has much to offer, so it's crucial to find out if your doctor can offer conventional treatment options. (Remember: you can always investigate your options and choose to say no to those treatment options. It's your body, your life.)

But what if you've seen five doctors, have a medical chart three inches thick, and in spite of everyone's best efforts, nobody has been able to figure out what's wrong with you? If you're one of those frustrated patients whom doctors haven't been able to give a diagnosis, don't despair. Sometimes your diagnosis is right around the corner, and it's just a matter of seeing the right physician. But other times, a conventional medical diagnosis simply doesn't exist, which is actually *great news*.

It's not that your symptoms are "all in your head," because clearly, they're in your body. But when you're experiencing symptoms your doctor can't diagnose, it's often because the symptoms are the result of repetitive triggering of the stress response without adequate relaxation-response counterbalancing. Conventional medicine simply doesn't yet have a catch-all diagnosis for that physiological cascade of symptom-inducing effects.

Whether you have a traditional diagnosis, you're experiencing symptoms nobody can diagnose, or you're healthy but interested in preventive health, chances are good that you're not optimizing your body's capacity for self-repair and improving your chance of cure. That's where the next step in this process comes in. Almost every illness is either caused by or exacerbated by triggering of the stress response, which happens in the body but starts in the mind. While you can mitigate some of the stress response without understanding what's triggering it, you're better off digging deep and diagnosing the root cause of *what is triggering those stress responses in the first place.* If you're engaging in stress-relieving activities, such as meditation, creative expression, sex, or exercise, but you're not alleviating the source of the stress, you're not optimizing your body's chance for cure. If, however, you can heal the problem from the root and stop the stress response at its origin, you're much more likely to wind up cured.

When you diagnose the root causes of what is triggering your stress responses, you gain insight into how your body may be suffering as the result of your mind and how you can not only prevent future stress responses but initiate natural relaxation responses that have been proven to prevent and cure disease. Remember, prevention is always better than treatment, especially given that some manifestations of chronic stress in the body may be hard (though not impossible) for the body to undo after the fact.

While it may be too late to prevent an illness that already affects you, it's never too late to reduce stress responses and activate relaxation responses. While results vary and some conditions are more susceptible than others to reductions in stress responses and increases in relaxation, when you mobilize the body's natural mechanisms of self-repair, anything is possible and spontaneous remission just might happen, even when you've been told your condition is chronic or incurable.

Before I move on to a series of exercises aimed at helping you identify what might be triggering your stress responses, let me say a few words about blame, shame, and guilt, which often come up any time you initiate a conversation about root causes of illness or suggest that people might have the power to heal themselves. When I tell you that you might have the power to heal yourself, and when you realize that something within your control may be causing or exacerbating a health condition, you may be inclined to either kick yourself or kick me. Since I'd prefer to avoid both outcomes, let me officially declare this a blame/shame/guilt-free zone.

Being sick doesn't mean you've necessarily done anything wrong. It also doesn't mean you're always the victim of sheer bad luck. Somewhere in the middle lies the truth. Clearly, there are dozens of factors that play into why one person gets sick and another doesn't or why one patient experiences spontaneous remission and another stays sick. Contributing factors include the beliefs of the conscious and subconscious mind, the right health-care providers, diet, self-care habits, feeling loved and worthy, being happy, practices that initiate the relaxation response, and spiritual factors I won't get into here.

Clearly you have a lot of control over how healthy you are. If you're a three-pack-a-day smoker who winds up with lung cancer, you've been eating at McDonald's every day and get a heart attack, you've been boozing it up for three decades and wind up with cirrhosis of the liver, or you've stayed in an abusive marriage for so long that you get an autoimmune disease, it's clear that your lifestyle choices are probably affecting the health of your body.

But things also happen to your body that are completely out of your control. You're born with an extra chromosome. Your car is hit by a drunk driver. You unwittingly move in next to a toxic-waste dump. You're the victim of a drive-by shooting. The rebounder trampoline you're bouncing on snaps closed while you're bouncing on it and breaks your wrist.

Shit happens.

Whether your illness came about because you smoked too much, drank too much, overate, or were just plain unlucky, there's no point berating yourself for past events you can't change. Doing so will only trigger stress responses and make things worse.

But there is a place for personal responsibility. As Dr. Christiane Northrup once said to me when we were discussing this issue, "We are responsible *to* our disease, not *for* our disease."

I agree with her. Illness offers us a precious opportunity to investigate our lives without judgment, diagnose the root cause of what might be contributing to an illness, realign ourselves spiritually, and do what we can to make our bodies ripe for miracles. When viewed with compassion and without judgment, illness can be a potent opportunity for personal growth and spiritual awakening.

Remember, before you go through these diagnostic exercises, make sure you have the right support. We're about to get down and dirty, and I want to make sure you feel safe, loved, and nurtured, not just by someone else, but especially by yourself. With that in mind, let me walk you through a few exercises I use with my patients to help them diagnose the root causes of what might be contributing to an illness.

Diagnostic Exercise #1:
What Does Your Body Need in Order to Heal?

1. Close your eyes and breathe deeply.

2. Tap into the wisdom of your Inner Pilot Light.

3. Ask yourself, "What does my body need in order to heal?" Your Inner Pilot Light might offer treatment intuitions—yes or no on a medication, for example. But I invite you to dig deeper. Beyond what your doctor is recommending, what *else* does your body need in order to heal? Be willing to tell yourself the truth.

4. With a nonjudgmental mind, spend 20 minutes listening quietly to what your Inner Pilot Light communicates to you. Remember, you don't have to take action on anything that comes up. The goal is simply to discover the truth about what your body needs in order to heal. Pull out your journal and write about it if you feel so inspired.

5. To download a guided meditation leading you through this process, visit MindOverMedicineBook.com.

Work/Life Balance

Although true work/life balance is almost impossible—many believe it's merely a crazy-making myth that leaves us striving for perfection and feeling chronically inadequate—it's important to be mindful of how we spend our time and whether we're prioritizing activities that induce the relaxation response. While finding the perfect balance between work life, family life, and personal life is challenging, and while I don't think it's always possible to have a balanced day, I do think it's possible to have a balanced week. I make a practice of switching out the radical self-care practices I wish I could do daily but don't always manage to fit in. For example, in a perfect world, my average day would start with waking up and meditating, practicing yoga, making a homemade batch of green juice, and preparing a healthy, organic breakfast to enjoy with my husband and daughter. Then I'd write, paint, attend to other work matters, have lunch with a friend, work some more, go for a hike, read to my daughter, cook another healthy meal for dinner, and end my day enjoying hot sex with my husband.

As if!

The reality is that some days I'm on a tight deadline and I work a 14-hour day, barely seeing my husband or daughter, skipping my meditation and hike, eating takeout, overlooking my creative pursuits, and barely managing to kiss my husband goodnight, much less rally for a little nookie. But I try to make that a rare occasion. And I try to balance it out. If I have a day like that on Monday, I do everything within my power to prioritize my family and my self-care on Tuesday, even if it means my work is delayed. By Wednesday, I look back over the week to see whether I've gotten in my meditation, exercised, eaten well, loved on my honey, spent quality time with my daughter, and allowed myself to create, all of which induce relaxation responses in me, nurture my mind and body, and keep me happy and healthy. By the end of the week, hopefully I've had a balanced week, even if I never got around to accomplishing all the work and self-care habits I aim to include as a regular part of my life.

The next exercise is designed to help you assess your work/life balance so you can get a feel for whether imbalances in your Whole Health Cairn may be harming your health. Pay attention to which stones in your Whole Health Cairn induce relaxation responses for you and which ones are stressors.

Diagnostic Exercise #2:
How Balanced Is Your Whole Health Cairn?

1. Photocopy seven copies of the Whole Health Cairn from this book (page 171) or print out copies you can download at MindOverMedicineBook.com.

2. Each day of the week, using crayons or markers, color in the stones in the Whole Health Cairn that you nurtured. For example, if you meditated, fill in your Spirituality stone. If you had good sex, fill in Sexuality. If you took good care of your physical body, fill in Physical Health. If you took time out to be a good mom or nurtured a relationship with your best friend, fill in your Relationships stone. If all you did was work, fill in your Work/Life Purpose stone . . . and so forth.

3. At the end of the week, pay attention to where you are focusing most of your time and energy. Are you skipping the same stones every day? Is your Whole Health Cairn out of balance? Which stones need attention?

Diagnose the Root Causes of Illness

The next exercise is designed to help you identify any limiting or self-sabotaging beliefs about your health, determine whether you feel supported by the right health-care providers, and use the Whole Health Cairn as a diagnostic tool to identify aspects of your life that might be triggering your stress responses and predisposing you to illness. It's also designed to help you get a feel for what activities in your life might elicit the relaxation response as part of your treatment. The goal of this exercise is to help you identify issues that are getting between you and optimal health.

Of all the steps in this six-step process, this one exercise is the most vital. It can also be the hardest. So please listen to your Inner Pilot Light as you work through this section. And call upon your support system.

Diagnostic Exercise #3:
Make the Diagnosis for Yourself

PART ONE

Ask yourself this series of questions, and be sure you go at your own speed. Take as much time as you need to answer the questions fully and honestly. And if you need to take a break or even stop, that's okay too. I can assure you that if you're willing to be truthful with yourself in answering the questions in this section, your Inner Pilot Light will grant you a precious gift—the opportunity to know what's true for you so you can make The Diagnosis for yourself.

You may want to talk through these questions out loud, by yourself or with a loved one. Or you may want to journal about them. To download The Diagnosis Journal, which leaves you room to write in the answers to the following questions, visit MindOverMedicineBook.com.

Try to be infinitely compassionate with yourself during this process. If you find yourself spiraling downward into negative thoughts, take a break, get support, and come back to it later with the help of your support system. Make sure to be radically nurturing with yourself. As you answer these questions, focus on gratitude, fill your life with pleasure, and be your own best friend. Doing so can ease the discomfort you may feel and keep you focusing on what's working in your life so you can be fearless enough to face and change what isn't.

BELIEF

- What do I believe about my genetics and how my genes affect my health?

- What are my beliefs about health?

- What are my beliefs about my illness?

- What are my beliefs about the body's ability to repair itself?

- What are my beliefs about my mind's effect on my body?

- Am I open to exploring that the root cause of my illness is not purely physical? If not, why not?

- What do I gain from my illness?

- Am I willing to give up what I gain from my illness in order to get well?

- Am I worthy of optimal health?

- How is my childhood affecting my current health?

SUPPORT

- How seen and heard do I feel by my health-care providers?

- What is my biggest fear about giving up a health-care provider?

- Am I asking for what I need from my health-care providers? If not, why not?

- Are there any ways I'm sabotaging my own health care?

- How do I support my own health?

- How do I feel when I leave my health-care provider?

- What would make me feel better supported in my relationship with my health-care providers?

- Am I fully disclosing what's true to my health-care provider? If not, why not?

- Am I worthy of having a close partnership with my health-care providers?

- What issues from my past might keep me from feeling able to partner with my health-care providers as an empowered patient?

INNER PILOT LIGHT

- Am I living an authentic life aligned with all that I desire?

- Do I make an effort to have my desires met?

- What does my Inner Pilot Light want me to know?

- When my intuition communicates with me, how much do I listen?

- What truth am I unwilling to face in my life right now?

- What within me am I holding back? What longs to be set free?

- What comes between me and my Inner Pilot Light?

- Am I willing to risk everything in order to listen to my Inner Pilot Light? If not, why not?

- Who would I be if I were fearless?

- On a scale of one to ten, how much do I love and accept myself?

RELATIONSHIPS

- How do I feel about my romantic life? How do I feel about my friends and support network?

- What are the repetitive relationship patterns that continue to appear in my life?

- Is there someone I need to forgive? Am I willing to forgive this person? Why or why not?

- How can I feel optimally loved?

- How vulnerable am I willing to be with the people in my life?

- What obituaries would I write if the people I love died today? If my loved ones were to die—or have already died—how much have I left unsaid?

- In the context of my relationships, is there always somebody wrong and somebody right?

- How often do I feel used in my relationships? Am I willing to release the victim or savior role in order to heal?

- Do I feel worthy of love and affection?

- What would I change about the love in my life if I had a magic wand?

WORK/LIFE PURPOSE

- What is true for me about my work?

- What does my Inner Pilot Light want me to know about my work?

- Is how I spend most of my day in line with my talents and purpose?

- What are my natural gifts?

- How does my body feel when I'm at work? How does my mind feel when I'm at work?

- If someone handed me a microphone and put me in front of an audience on the last day of my life, what would I say to the world?

- If all my financial needs were met and the needs of my family were met, what would I do with my time?

- If I took fear out of the equation, what would I change about how I spend my days?

- Is my job the bridge to getting me where I want to go?

- Am I learning valuable things in my day job that I'm supposed to know, even if I don't love the work I do?

CREATIVITY

- What lights my creative fire? Who or what is my muse?

- Am I clear on what my soul wants to create?

- What helps my creativity flow freely?

- What kinds of creative projects light me up? Am I doing these things regularly?

- What creative projects did I engage in as a child?

- If I had all the time and money in the world, what would I create?

- How do I feel when I don't feel inspired?

- Am I willing to be with the frustration of the creative process?

- Do I feel worthy of expressing myself creatively?

- What does my family believe about creativity?

SPIRITUALITY

- What makes me feel spiritually connected?

- What do I consider sacred?

- If I don't consider myself "religious" or even believe in a Higher Power, am I finding other ways to nurture my spiritual self?

- What are my thoughts and feelings about religion? What negative thoughts do I have about spirituality or religion?

- Do I feel more spiritual in a spiritual community, or am I more of a loner when it comes to my spiritual life?

- Am I open to letting illness be an opportunity for spiritual awakening?

- What does my family believe about spirituality?

- Are there ways in which I use my spirituality or religion to judge others?

- Am I worthy of experiencing a deep connection with the Divine?

- Would joining the right spiritual community elicit relaxation responses in my body?

SEXUALITY

- What do I truly desire sexually? Am I fulfilling that desire?

- What will help support my authentic sexual self?

- What fears, beliefs, or hang-ups keep me from being as sexually honest and openly expressed as I might wish to be?

- How do I feel about my first sexual experience?

- What from my sexual past or present life may be in need of healing?

- What *really* turns me on? What *really* turns me off?

- How do I feel about having sex when I don't want to?

- Do I feel sensual when I'm not having sex?

- What does my family believe about sexuality?

- If I could do anything sexually and nobody else ever had to know, what would I do?

MONEY

- What are my thoughts and feelings about my financial situation?

- How financially healthy am I?

- How do I define financial health, success, or abundance?

- Am I clear about the true state of my financial life, or have I buried my head in the sand?

- What does my family believe about money?

- What limiting beliefs about my finances do I need to release?

- Do I have enough money to support me in case of an emergency?

- Is it possible to be poor and happy?

- How much time do I spend thinking about money?

- Does money buy me love?

ENVIRONMENT

- Am I living where my Inner Pilot Light wants to live?

- When I look around at my surroundings, do I love what I see?

- Am I surrounded by beauty? Does my environment include nature?

- How healthy is my environment?

- What environmental exposures might be affecting my health?

- On a scale of 1 to 10, how "green" am I?

- What efforts do I make to reduce the toxic load on my body caused by my environment?

- What environmental exposures might be affecting my health?

- How might I eliminate unnecessary clutter from my environment?

- Do I feel worthy of living in a healing, peaceful environment I love?

MENTAL HEALTH

- What makes me happy? What makes me unhappy?

- What would heal my mind?

- Do any traumas from my past still cause me suffering? If so, what are they?

- Do I feel worthy of being happy?

- How much time do I spend engaging in negative conversations such as unkind gossip, criticism of another person, or complaining?

- Am I willing to examine my mental health?

- What am I grateful for?

- Do I express gratitude for what I appreciate in my life on a regular basis?

- What can I be grateful for today?

- Do I get caught up in what I lack rather than appreciating what I have?

PHYSICAL HEALTH

- How are my diet and exercise habits?

- How compliant am I with my health-care provider's recommendations and protocols?

- What bad habits do I need to release?

- How are my energy levels?

- Is anything keeping me from sleeping well?

- How much do I prioritize my physical health?

- Am I willing to invest time, money, and energy in taking better care of my body?

- What will happen to me if my body is optimally healthy? How will others feel about it?

- How do I feel about aging?

- How do I feel about death?

WRAP-UP

- How much am I willing to fully accept myself in all my divine imperfections?

- How much permission do I give myself to make mistakes?

- Am I willing to fiercely love and accept myself during my healing journey?

- After answering these questions, does my Inner Pilot Light feel illuminated? Do I feel I have everything I need in order to make my body ripe for miracles?

- Am I willing to use what I've learned to write The Prescription for myself and make changes in my life?

PART TWO

Using the answers to these questions, can you identify the root causes associated with your illness? Are negative beliefs sabotaging you? Do you have the right support? Are there any issues in your Whole Health Cairn that might be triggering your stress responses and harming your body? Are there activities that would elicit relaxation responses in your body that you're not utilizing? Have these questions helped illuminate any blind spots in your life you needed to see in order to be optimally healthy?

Within each category, write down in The Diagnosis Journal, which you can download at MindOverMedicineBook.com, anything you've identified that you believe is benefiting your health and that you might want to ramp up in your life as part of a plan of radical self-care.

Congratulations! You just made The Diagnosis. What you just listed are your interpretations of what may be harming and benefiting your health. To read The Diagnosis I wrote for myself before most of my health issues resolved, see Appendix B.

STEP FIVE: Write the Prescription for Yourself

Now that you've chosen to listen to your body, tapped into the wisdom of your Inner Pilot Light, investigated your beliefs and your support team, evaluated what might be out of balance in your Whole Health Cairn, and diagnosed any underlying causes that might be harming your health, it's time to make a whole-health treatment plan of radical self-care.

When you get sick, your doctor may prescribe a different kind of treatment plan. For example, if you get cancer and you have a smart, savvy, holistic physician, your treatment plan may include surgery, chemotherapy, a nourishing raw-food or vegan diet, a host of supplements meant to ramp up your immune system, a support group to help you deal with the emotions of cancer, and a yoga practice to keep you centered.

That kind of treatment plan will get you far. But if the root cause of your weakened immune system is loneliness, job stress, or depression, treating the cancer without treating the root causes may help in the short term, but it may not be permanent. The cancer may come back—or you'll wind up with some other illness. In order to optimally prevent and treat disease so you don't keep circling back to a weakened, sick body, you must, must, *must* address the root causes that make you susceptible to illness in the first place, while listening to your Inner Pilot Light and letting it help you choose how to maximize what conventional medicine has to offer in a way that is in alignment for you.

That's what writing The Prescription is all about.

Part of writing The Prescription for yourself is stepping up to the plate as the head honcho of your health care. Remember, you're the boss. Everyone else is in service to you.

Sure, your doctor will order lab tests and help you diagnose what's wrong. Your doctor will write prescriptions for any drugs you need. If you need surgery or some other medical procedure, your doctor will handle that too. But it's *up to you* whether you take those drugs or submit to that surgery. That's what writing The Prescription for yourself means. You don't just blindly obey doctor's orders. You become a full partner in the healing process. You check in with your body, listen to your Inner Pilot Light, and consult the people you invite to sit at the healing round table with you.

When you're making decisions about your health care, go ahead and consult with the best but remember that *they are there to serve you*. Invite to the healing round table your doctor, your therapist, your acupuncturist, your massage therapist, your life coach, your mother—whoever! They're your steering committee, your advisory board, your educators.

Pick them wisely. If you can afford it, be willing to pay extra to choose the best people you can get to your healing round table. But never forget that it's your table. The seat of honor is reserved for you. The people at your table may disagree with each other. It's possible you'll get confused by opposing opinions. But stand your ground. You know your body better than anyone else.

If there were only one right way to heal the body, we'd all agree. But there's not. That's why they call it the art of medicine. Ultimately, the treatment plan has to feel right to you. It's your body. Your life. Your choice. You always get the deciding vote. When you listen to the inner knowing that comes from deep connection to your Inner Pilot Light and your body, you'll always make the right choices for you.

Writing The Prescription for yourself doesn't stop at picking the right health-care team and being an active participant in the treatment plan. It goes deeper. Perhaps what you've learned in this book has led you to realize that your limiting, self-sabotaging, negative beliefs about your health are translating into bad news for your body. Perhaps you've realized that loneliness is hurting your body. Perhaps you had an aha moment when you read the data about how work stress can kill you. Maybe you realized that it's time to convert from pessimism to optimism and ramp up your happiness. Or maybe the Whole Health Cairn helped you identify some imbalances in your life that might be affecting your health.

Here's where you get to translate your new awareness into an action plan. I don't want you to just *know* why you might not be optimally healthy. I want you to *do* something about it, and only you know best what that something will be. Your doctor might be able to prescribe your pills, but only *you* can write The Prescription for how your life needs to change in order to optimize your whole health.

Here's how you can get started.

A Therapeutic Exercise:
Write the Prescription for Yourself

1. Grab a pen and pull out a few sheets of paper or your journal, or download The Prescription form from MindOverMedicineBook.com.

2. Pull out The Diagnosis you've created for yourself on sheets of paper, in your journal, or in The Diagnosis Journal you downloaded.

3. Take a moment to close your eyes and tap into the healing wisdom of your Inner Pilot Light. Remind yourself to stay open, loving, and compassionate with yourself. When you feel centered, relaxed, and intuitively open, open your eyes.

4. For each of the items you listed in The Diagnosis, ask yourself what you can do to take action in order to treat any root cause of illness you've identified. Trust your intuition and try not to judge what comes up. Remember, you don't have to actually implement these action steps yet, but you do have to be honest with yourself. Don't censor anything. *Nobody ever has to read this but you.*

5. Although much of my one-on-one work with patients includes specific recommendations for what my patients might include in The Prescription, those kinds of specific recommendations are beyond the scope of this book. For example, if you're having problems in your marriage, there are specific books I would recommend, therapists I trust, and workshops I would suggest. But the truth is, you'll be surprised how much you already know. You really don't need me or anyone else to tell you what your body—and your life—needs.

6. If you've identified an issue but aren't sure how to heal it, I won't leave you hanging. Follow my blog at LissaRankin .com, where I write practical prescriptions for living and loving fearlessly, as well as other techniques for healing yourself and living your best life. You can also check out OwningPink.com, where more than 30 healers and visionary teachers write about how to heal every stone in the Whole Health Cairn.

For a sample of The Prescription I wrote for myself, see Appendix C.

Take Action

Once you've written The Prescription, your journey is just beginning, because the next step in the process is the most exciting and requires the most courage. Once you know what changes you need to make in your life in order to optimize your health, it's time to take action.

Let me start with a little cheerleading. You can do this! I know, because I speak from personal experience. I remember vividly what it felt like to know—just *know*—what I had to do to save my life. And I was terrified. But I was also excited, because I knew in my heart of hearts that my life was about to change for the better.

I know the same is true for you, and I am here wildly waving pom-poms. Go you! I'm super proud of you already, just for drawing a line in the sand and stepping fearlessly over it.

I know your heart is probably racing. You might have butterflies. You might even trigger stress responses just thinking about how you'll muster up the nerve to face The Diagnosis and implement what you've written in The Prescription. But don't worry. Those are temporary. I promise the relaxation process follows soon afterward.

Having stepped out of traditional clinical practice to mentor clients through this process, I know how scary it is to do this, and I'm in constant awe of the fortitude of the human spirit. The massive changes I've witnessed in those brave enough to forge ahead on a healing journey like this have opened my heart and blown my mind. I've witnessed medical miracles—spontaneous remissions I can only explain as feats of physiological self-repair. I've always watched people face their fears, open their hearts, and transform their whole lives.

As you move forward, keep checking in with your Inner Pilot Light. Let your Inner Pilot Light be your best friend, constantly reminding you of the truth you seek and the knowing you trust. Your Inner Pilot Light will offer you infinite compassion during this process. The more you tap in, the more joyous this process can be.

But what if you're not willing to take action? What if you know what it will take to get well and you just can't take the leap of faith? If that's you, be kind to yourself. Maybe it's not time yet. Remember, you'll know when it's time to take a leap of faith when the pain of staying put exceeds the fear of the unknown. If you're not there yet, it's okay to wait.

But don't wait too long. I don't want your body to start screaming just because you're not willing to listen to the whispers.

For most people, making The Diagnosis and writing The Prescription command radical change, and some people simply aren't willing to act on what their Inner Pilot Lights are guiding them to do. The question I always ask patients is, "If you're not willing to take action, are you choosing to be sick?"

Some lower their eyes sheepishly and nod, admitting that they'd rather risk their health than face up to what they know needs to change. And that's okay. No judgment here. But it's good to 'fess up to the choices you make in life.

Others tell me they're willing to do anything, risk anything, brave anything, if there's even a sliver of hope that making the change will alter their physiology. These are the people who touch my heart and leave me misty. These are also the people who disproportionately get better.

Ultimately, it's your call. Your body. Your life.

Once you know what needs to change in your life and you decide you're going to go for it, be exceedingly compassionate with yourself. Go easy. Take baby steps. Reward yourself often. Serve yourself a heaping helping of acceptance, gratitude, and love. You'll need it to fuel your journey.

STEP SIX: Surrender Attachment to Outcomes

There comes a time, after you've shifted to positive belief, found the right support, tapped into the wisdom of your body and your Inner Pilot Light, made The Diagnosis, written The Prescription, and taken action on it, to simply surrender and let go of attaching to any particular outcome. Yes, you want to be cured. Who doesn't when they're sick? But the truth is that it might not happen. And it's not your fault.

I believe that while we hold within us the power to make changes in our life designed to foster the body's ability to self-repair, we must accept that, when it comes right down to it, we have no guarantees as to whether or not we will stay sick or get well. You can do everything "right" and still wind up dying. In fact, it's guaranteed that we will all face this inevitable fate at some point in our lives. You can also do nothing and experience spontaneous remission.

Too often, those who make a radical commitment to self-healing feel like failures if their diseases don't disappear. But why go there? Who are we to know what the Universe has in store for us? How can we anticipate what lessons we're here on this earth to learn and what life challenges we need to face in order to learn them? Perhaps some of us are meant to be sick so we can learn what our soul longs to learn and model how to weather illness with grace. The grace comes in fighting until it's time to stop fighting, and appreciating every step of the journey, even when it doesn't go our way.

It's hard to anticipate how you will feel about your self-healing journey, so I want to give you a little heads-up. Having supported the self-healing journeys of many people, I can attest to the fact that the journey is different for everyone, and outcomes vary. For example, one of my patients had been suffering from a chronic illness for 20 years when we started working through this process together. After three months of regular sessions and intense work on her part, her disease vanished. I was thrilled! It worked!

But she was grief-stricken, barely able to get out of bed every morning, even though her physical symptoms were completely gone. Mourning the 20 years she felt she had lost from a disease she now realized she could have cured solely with the power of her mind, she spun into depression until a daily gratitude practice, an opportunity to serve those less fortunate than her, and the birth of her grandson pulled her out of her despair. Her experience helped me realize how important it is to live in the present when you're going through a process like this. Remaining optimistic, focusing on gratitude, and appreciating what you have is vital to keep you from spinning out into regrets and sadness about what might have been. If you're blessed to experience a spontaneous remission as the result of this process, please, I beg of you, thank your lucky stars and say prayers of thanks. You were blessed with a second chance, and you have an opportunity to take what you've learned and use it to help others.

Another patient of mine who experienced spontaneous remission had the complete opposite experience. Although she too had suffered from her illness, she never once looked back when her illness was cured. She viewed her cure as a miracle that opened her up to a richer spiritual life and transformed not just her health but her romantic life, her professional life, and where she lived.

Yet another patient worked through this whole process with such courage, even in the face of rapidly declining health. She fearlessly faced her truth; realigned all sorts of relationship contracts in her life; started living her dream; released old resentments; let go of old, stale fears; forgave people she had been holding grudges against since childhood; released herself from the false identity of her ego; and aligned with her Inner Pilot Light in every aspect of her life. Although she ultimately succumbed to her illness, she did so with such grace that her death was a healing to dozens of other people, especially her family. She wasn't cured, but she died healed. Hundreds showed up for her funeral to express their gratitude for a life well lived and well ended.

What more can we hope for as we navigate this journey? It's a win-win situation. Whether or not you're cured, you will be healed, and your healing will offer a healing to others.

I encourage you to remember that it will be a rebirth, if you're open to experiencing it, and on the other side, you will expand in ways you may not even be able to imagine. Surrendering attachment to outcomes when you're sick, after you've done everything within your power to make your body ripe for miracles, allows illness to be an opportunity for spiritual awakening. If you let it, being sick can blast your ego, light a fire under you to reprioritize your life, remind you to appreciate what you have, align your life with your Inner Pilot Light, give you the courage to live in the moment, and bring you closer to loved ones and to the Divine.

When I did an art project I called "The Woman Inside Project," during which I cast the torsos of women with breast cancer using medical-grade plaster, while interviewing them about the beauty that lies within them, almost every woman whose body I sculpted said cancer was the best thing that ever happened to her because it led her to take steps in her life that turned out to effect lasting positive change.

We shouldn't have to wait for illness to realign with our truth, but often we do. Just like I needed my Perfect Storm to wake up, many need to get sick so they get jolted out of their complacency and start living as if they might die tomorrow.

If illness strikes, it's a potent opportunity to wake up, even if part of what we're here to learn and teach is how to die with grace. While I believe miracles are always possible, sometimes a cure simply doesn't happen. We must make peace with this fact. If you set upon a quest to heal yourself while attaching to the outcome of complete cure, and then you find yourself still sick, you may wind up pitched into the despair of the dark night of the soul. But if you do everything within your power to make your body ripe for miracles—and *then you let go and trust the journey*—you pave the way for peace, serenity, and joy beyond your wildest imagining.

When You're Healed but Not Cured

I know. I witnessed it in my father.

When my father got sick with a brain tumor that wound up being metastatic melanoma, Dad believed he would beat it. He was young—too young—and he was an optimist with great faith, a supportive community, a family that adored him, and a wide-open heart. Dad certainly didn't do anything wrong to earn his cancer. He was a wonderful man who led a blessed life.

But he died anyway. It felt so unfair.

In the midst of researching this book, I was sitting with my mother on the six-year anniversary of Dad's death. Mom and I had been talking about what I was learning, and she asked me whether I thought Dad had done something wrong. Did he not believe enough in the possibility of remission? Did he not find the right support? Did he fail to balance his Whole Health Cairn? Should we have put him on a macrobiotic diet? Could Dad's death have been prevented?

I told her I honestly didn't know.

I've learned a lot in the process of researching and writing this book, and yet there is much I still don't know. Was Dad's death from cancer preventable? Might he have staved off the cancer if he drank green juice instead of eating chicken wings? Could he have saved himself by finding a new purpose after his early disability from multiple sclerosis led him to premature retirement? Might he have been cured if he had found a creative hobby that lit him up? Did Dad need more sex? Hours in meditation? A healthier environment? More laughter? More sunshine? Fewer stress responses? More relaxation responses?

It's impossible to say.

Maybe Dad could have been cured if he shifted his mind-set, found the right support, tapped into his Inner Pilot Light, made his own diagnosis, wrote The Prescription for himself, and took action.

But maybe not. Maybe he'd have done all that and the outcome would have been the same.

I hugged Mom and mused about what my father would think about this book if he had read it. The whole time I researched it, his voice was the voice in the back of my head, questioning me, prodding me, pushing me to go deeper, serving as the ultimate skeptic I was trying to win over.

I finally got up the nerve to ask my mother what she thought. If Dad were still alive, what would he think about what I was learning and writing about?

Mom was quiet and reflective. A tear formed in the corner of one eye. Then she smiled a crooked, sweet smile and told me that at first, he would have thought I'd gone off the deep end. But at some point, I would have appealed to the scientist in him. In the end, she suspected that even Dad would have looked at the evidence, compelled to open his mind *just enough* to consider that maybe there was at least a grain of truth here.

When she said that, I started to cry.

"What I do know for sure," Mom said, "is that, if your father were here right now, he'd be incredibly proud."

In that moment, I missed my father so much that I could feel my heart, right under my left breast, hollow and raw and sore and at the same time, full and overflowing. I confessed to Mom that I wrote this whole book to my father. His were the eyes on the other side of the page as I wrote. Perhaps if I could write a book that even doctors like my father could read without instantly shooing it away, maybe I could make a real difference in how health care is received and delivered. Maybe I could serve out my calling to redefine health and help people heal in a whole new way. Maybe I could attract a tribe of doctors and patients and other health-care providers who know our system is broken and long to reclaim the heart of medicine. Maybe I could teach people how to take responsibility for their health and bring the sacred back to the practice of medicine. Maybe—just maybe—I could help heal my beloved profession.

As the fictional physician character in Dr. Abraham Verghese's *Cutting for Stone* states, "We come unbidden into this life, and if we are lucky, we find a purpose beyond starvation, misery, and early death which, lest we forget, is the common lot. I grew up and I found my purpose, and it was to become a physician. My intent wasn't to save the world as much as to heal myself. Few doctors will admit this, certainly not young ones, but subconsciously, in entering the profession, we must believe that ministering to others will heal our woundedness. And it can. But it can also deepen the wound."

I was one of those doctors for whom the wound was deepened, and it made my body sick. But now, having learned how to heal myself, I long to help others do the same. The biggest lesson I've learned is that you can spend your life running scared and clinging to the illusion of control, grasping for what you think is certain until your life—and your health—suddenly crumble around you. Or you can recognize that the only thing certain in life is uncertainty. Whether you fear uncertainty and let it trigger stress responses or embrace uncertainty and let it elicit relaxation responses is your choice. Personally, I've come to recognize the beauty in uncertainty. While one face of uncertainty is the vast, scary unknown, the flip side of uncertainty is infinite possibility. When you don't know what the future holds, anything can happen.

These days, when I wake up in the morning, I'm fully aware that I have no idea what lies before me. Sure, I have a calendar filled with events, but events change, new opportunities arise, and my schedule has become fluid. What I thought I would be doing this year is different than what I anticipated a year ago. In fact, it's better than anything I could have even dreamed. Which is good news. It means that next year could hold even more gems I don't yet know to include in my fantasies. The world is my oyster. The sky's the limit. Look out, world.

The same is true for you. While you may feel fearful because you don't know what the future holds (especially if you're sick), anything could happen to you tomorrow. You could go to sleep tonight sick and wake up cured. Your symptoms could disappear forever. Your mood could lift. The love of your life could be standing behind you in Starbucks. The deal could come through. The house of your dreams could land in your lap. Oprah could call. You could finally get pregnant. You could win the lottery. Your long-lost mother could show up. You could find enlightenment. The seas could part in front of your very eyes.

If you are well and you've gone through these steps as a way to prevent disease in your life, high-five to you! I applaud you for your courage and firmly believe you've just extended your life. And if you've done this because you're sick, high-fives to you too!

This is your precious life. Savor it. Grab the ring on the carousel. Ride the roller coaster. Do cartwheels. Open your heart. Never leave love unexpressed. Forgive generously. Give openly. Follow your dream. Speak your truth. Laugh at fear. Take leaps of faith. Make beautiful things. Honor what you desire. Experience pleasure. Let your freak flag fly. Live daringly. Be unapologetically you. It's preventive medicine. And it just might save your life.

Appendix A

8 TIPS FOR HOW TO BE IN YOUR BODY

- **Focus on a body part.** Notice your right fingertip or your left knee or any other body part. How does it feel? Does it hurt? Is it cool or warm? Do you feel a breeze? Notice how it feels when you stroke it with a feather or brush it against the carpet. Pay attention to all your senses.

- **Name your sensation.** Although words come from the mind, they can help connect the mind and the body by giving a name to what you feel. Be specific with the words you choose— does your body part feel stiff, loose, light, heavy, tingly, warm, cold, sensitive, numb, strong, weak, painful? Try to avoid describing your sensation in general terms such as "good" or "bad." Perhaps you feel clenched or spacious or prickly or heavy. Be as multisensory as you can.

- **Practice movement.** Dancing, yoga, hiking, cycling, skiing, and other such physical activity can make you more aware of your body—what feels yummy and what hurts! Even pain can be a teacher about body awareness, so don't be afraid to lean into what you feel.

- **Use the floor.** If you're having trouble feeling your body in space, try rolling around on the floor. It gives your body something to be in relationship with.

- **Optimize clothing.** Wearing loose-fitting clothes that brush against your skin when you move can help you notice your body. If you wear tight-fitting clothes, you may notice your body less than if you wear free-flowing pants or skirts and shirts with loose sleeves.

- **Get sexual.** Nothing like a good romp in the hay to help you notice your body!

- **When trying to make a decision, notice how your body is responding.** That guy who asked you out? How does your body feel—light or heavy? New job offer? Does your body feel open or closed? Your body is your compass. Pay attention.

- **Breathe.** When you pay attention to your breathing, it helps center you in your body.

Appendix B

LISSA'S PERSONAL
SELF-HEALING DIAGNOSIS

These are the areas of my life I diagnosed as being out of alignment with my optimal health before I began implementing The Prescription I wrote for myself.

BELIEF

- I don't believe I can heal myself because I was taught to revere conventional medicine and turn over my power to physicians.

SUPPORT

- I need to go outside conventional medicine to find the people to invite to my healing round table.

INNER PILOT LIGHT

- I've covered up so much of myself with masks in order to make myself acceptable to others that I don't even know who I am anymore. My Inner Pilot Light feels like it's completely burned out, but I know it's there.

- I feel dissociated from my body. I want to hear the whispers of my body before my body screams.

RELATIONSHIPS

- The death of my father is harming my health. I need to grieve.

- Sometimes I feel lonely. I'm surrounded by people, but I feel like so many of them don't see or know the real me.

- I love my husband, but I want to feel closer to him to safeguard against failing in marriage *again.*

- I give until I'm depleted.

WORK/LIFE PURPOSE

- My work is trying to kill me.

- I have no idea what my life purpose is anymore.

CREATIVITY

- I feel creatively intoxicated and sense that it's a crucial part of my healing process. More, please.

- I love writing but don't do it enough. I think more writing would benefit my health.

SPIRITUALITY

- I wish I felt closer to God and think it would benefit my health, but the religion in which I was raised just isn't me.

- I still pray, and I think that helps my health.

SEXUALITY

- I think a more fulfilling sex life would benefit my health.

MONEY

- I earn a good living and feel financially secure but at what price? My job is draining me.

- If I quit, I'll be broke, and that stresses me out.

ENVIRONMENT

- Southern California has gotten so busy and crowded that I feel stressed out where I live. I live so close to my neighbors I can pass eggs to them over the balcony.

- I long for more nature, space, and serenity in my living environment. I wish I could move to Big Sur. I think that would be good for my health.

MENTAL HEALTH

- I'm not clinically depressed and am inclined to be optimistic and cheerful, but I have this deep underlying sadness I can't shake, maybe left over from my failed marriage, my grueling medical education, and all the loved ones I've lost. I think taking steps to optimize my happiness would benefit my health.

PHYSICAL HEALTH

- Although my diet is pretty good at home, work keeps me so busy that I'm not eating well at work.

- Even my diet at home could be better. I eat *way* too much cheese.

- I don't exercise as much as I used to because my pregnancy left me with a bum hip. I think more exercise would be good for my health.

- I'd probably be healthier if I lost the 20 pounds I've put on in the past few years.

- I hate taking seven medications for all these health issues, but I'm compliant with my regimen and that helps my health.

Appendix C

LISSA'S PERSONAL PRESCRIPTION

BELIEF

- Eliminate limiting belief by working with EFT practitioners Kate Winch and Nick Ortner to practice Emotional Freedom Technique (EFT).

- Do body-centered therapy sessions with Steve Sisgold aimed at changing beliefs in my body.

- Do a Psych-K session with Rita Somen.

SUPPORT

- Gather my healing round table of practitioners from many disciplines.

INNER PILOT LIGHT

- Commit to stripping off the masks and being unapologetically ME in all aspects of my life.

- Schedule time at retreat centers like Esalen Institute and Kripalu.

- Learn to get into my body with Nia Technique, a sensory-based movement practice taught by Debbie Rosas.

- Get an astrological reading with Ophira Edut of the AstroTwins.

RELATIONSHIPS

- Put into practice the "gifts of imperfection" taught by Brené Brown in her books and TEDx and TED talks. Be willing to be vulnerable, expose my flaws, and allow deeper intimacy through the connections that results when I give up the impossible quest for perfection.

- Stop trying to *save* everyone I love. Love them unconditionally just the way they are, but resist the urge to fix them.

- Heal my "savior complex." Commit to filling myself first, so I'm full enough to help others.

- Make a list of the people I want to be mindful of every day so I can make sure I'm a good friend to the people I love. Put the list on my altar and look at it daily.

- Stop expecting people to read my mind and fully communicate what I want and need in my relationships. Ask others to be equally forthright with what they want and need from me.

- Be mindful of the often unconscious agreements I make with people. Trade in unspoken agreements for conscious sacred contracts both parties agree to uphold.

- Follow the advice of Martha Beck and make a list of all the people whose opinions I really value and then let go of caring about what *everybody* who is not on the list thinks.

- See others with "magical eyes" (soul to soul).

WORK/LIFE PURPOSE

- Quit my conventional medicine job.

- Overcome my resistance to my calling to help heal my profession and change how health care is received and delivered.

- Heal myself from the pain I experienced in my profession with Dr. Rachel Naomi Remen and her community of healing M.D.'s.

- Launch OwningPink.com, a web community where those in need of healing can connect with those committed to healing others, where both patients and healers can find resources to help them thrive.

- Launch my solo blog at LissaRankin.com.

- Read everything Martha Beck ever wrote.

- Hire Melanie Bates, the perfect virtual assistant/editor/coach to lift up my business.

- Learn to claim my power and leadership skills with leadership consultant Dana Theus.

- Join a mastermind group with fellow authors/coaches like Amy Ahlers, Mike Robbins, Christine Arylo, and Steve Sisgold.

CREATIVITY

- Develop creativity rituals, such as meditating at my creativity altar, lighting a candle, and saying my daily prayer.

- Write blog posts at LissaRankin.com and OwningPink.com.

- Practice writing from the heart in a workshop with Nancy Aronie, author of *Writing from the Heart.*

- Do studio visits with 60 inspiring artists in order to write my book *Encaustic Art: The Complete Guide to Creating Fine Art with Wax.*

- Write more.

- Paint whenever possible.

- Create multi-media e-courses (available at LissaRankin.com).

SPIRITUALITY

- Meditate for at least 20 minutes per day.

- Seek wisdom and guidance from intuitive spiritual counselor Tricia Barrett.

- Attend dharma talks at Green Gulch Zen Center and Spirit Rock Meditation Center.

- Pray daily and ask to receive and know how to interpret signs from the Universe that guide my path.

- Spend time tending to my personal altar.

SEXUALITY

- Take sensual feminine movement classes at Sheila Kelley's S Factor.

- Graduate from Mama Gena's School of Womanly Arts Mastery program with Regena Thomashauer.

- Learn how to OM (Orgasmic Meditation) with Nicole Daedone of One Taste.

- Experiment with some other hot stuff I'll choose to keep secret.

MONEY

- Repeat affirmations and practice EFT to end limiting beliefs I have about money.

- Work with financial coach Barbara Stanny to release limiting beliefs about money.

- Make a budget (finally).

- Get clear on my financial goals. Set intentions. Release fears related to money. Trust the process.

ENVIRONMENT

- Leave city living in Southern California.

- Realize that things don't equal happiness and start decluttering my life. Start with my clothes closet.

- Feng shui my house to create a more healing environment.

- Make efforts to green my home.

- Surround myself with the medicine of redwoods, mountains, and the ocean in coastal Northern California.

MENTAL HEALTH

- Recognize that pain is inevitable but suffering is optional. Consciously choose joy.

- Learn how to be more optimistic.

- Make gratitude a practice by going around the dinner table with my family every night and saying what we're all grateful for that day.

- Keep a gratitude journal.

- Unapologetically pursue what brings me pleasure, as long as it aligns with my integrity.

- Dance. Often. To loud music.

- Do cartwheels. Whenever the urge strikes. Just because it feels good.

- Indulge in homemade raw chocolate.

- Silence my inner critic (the Gremlin) and replace it with the voice of my Inner Pilot Light.

PHYSICAL HEALTH

- Drink green juice every day and do a detox cleanse every three months. (To try the cleanse I do, go to JuiceDietCleanse.com.)

- Follow my "raw vegan omnivore" diet (mostly veggies, mostly vegan, often raw, mostly gluten-free and sugar-free but with rare gourmet indulgences like duck, cheese, paninis, and crème brulée). Get inspiration from Kris Carr's book *Crazy Sexy Diet*.

- Cut back from three high-blood-pressure medications to half the dose of one.

- Stop all allergy pills, inhalers, and shots. Believe that I can heal myself from my allergies.

- See my conventional medical doctors, as well as a naturopathic doctor.

- Take daily vitamins (a multivitamin/antioxidant, calcium, a chelated mineral supplement, Vitamin D, and fish oil). Supplement my diet with chia seeds and sun chlorella.

- Hike or do yoga at least an hour per day.

- Sleep at least seven hours a night.

Continue Your Self-Healing Journey

To download a free Self-Healing Kit designed by Lissa Rankin to support your healing journey, visit MindOverMedicineBook.com.

ENDNOTES

Introduction

1. Anne Harrington, *The Cure Within: A History of Mind-Body Medicine* (New York: W. W. Norton & Company, 2008), 250–51.

2. Patrick Cooke, "They Cried until They Could Not See," *New York Times Magazine*, June 23, 1991.

Chapter 1

1. Bruno Klopfer, "Psychological Variables in Human Cancer," *Journal of Projective Techniques* 21, no. 4 (December 1957): 331–40.

2. Stewart Wolf, "The Effects of Suggestion and Conditioning on the Action of Chemical Agents in Human Subjects: The Pharmacology of Placebos," *Journal of Clinical Investigation* 29, no. 1 (January 1950): 100–109.

3. J. Bruce Moseley et al., "A Controlled Trial of Arthroscopic Surgery for Osteoarthritis of the Knee," *New England Journal of Medicine* 347 (July 11, 2002): 81–88.

4. Margaret Talbot, "The Placebo Prescription," *New York Times Magazine*, January 9, 2000.

5. Henry K. Beecher, "The Powerful Placebo," *Journal of the American Medical Association* 159, no. 17 (December 24, 1955): 1602–6.

6. Michael E. Wechsler et al., "Active Albuterol or Placebo, Sham Acupuncture, or No Intervention in Asthma," *New England Journal of Medicine* 365 (July 14, 2011): 119–26.

7. Femke M. de Groot et al., "Headache: The Placebo Effects in the Control Groups in Randomized Clinical Trials; An Analysis of Systematic Reviews," *Journal of Manipulative and Physiological Therapeutics* 34, no. 5 (June 2011): 297–305.

8. Talbot, "The Placebo Prescription."

9. H. J. Binder et al., "Cimetidine in the Treatment of Duodenal Ulcer: A Multicenter Double Blind Study," *Gastroenterology* 74 (February 1978): 380–88.

10. Shirley S. Wang, "Why Placebos Work Wonders," *Wall Street Journal*, January 10, 2012, http://online.wsj.com/article/SB10001424052970204720204577128873886471982.html.

11. F. J. Evans, "Expectancy, Therapeutic Instructions, and the Placebo Response," in *Placebo: Theory, Research and Mechanisms*, ed. Leonard White, Bernard Tursky, and Gary E. Schwartz (New York: Guilford Press, 1985); J. D. Levine et al., "Analgesic Responses to Morphine and Placebo in Individuals with Postoperative Pain," *Pain* 10, no. 3 (June 1981): 379–89.

12. Irving Kirsch, *The Emperor's New Drugs: Exploding the Antidepressant Myth* (New York: Basic Books, 2010); Irving Kirsch and Guy Sapirstein, "Listening to Prozac but Hearing Placebo: A Meta-Analysis of Antidepressant Medication," *Prevention & Treatment* 1, no. 2 (June 1998); Shankar Vedantam, "Against Depression, a Sugar Pill Is Hard to Beat: Placebos Improve Mood, Change Brain Chemistry in Majority of Trials of Antidepressants," *Washington Post*, May 7, 2002; Arif Khan et al., "Suicide Rates in Clinical Trials of SSRIs, Other Antidepressants, and Placebo: Analysis of FDA Reports," *American Journal of Psychiatry* 160, no. 4 (April 1, 2003): 790–92.

13. Judith A. Turner et al., "The Importance of Placebo Effects in Pain Treatment and Research," *Journal of the American Medical Association* 271, no. 20 (May 25, 1994): 1609–14; Leonard A. Cobb et al., "An Evaluation of Internal-Mammary-Artery Ligation by a Double-Blind Technic," *New England Journal of Medicine*, 260, no. 22 (May 28, 1959): 1115–18.

14. Elise A. Olsen et al., "A Multicenter, Randomized, Placebo-Controlled, Double-Blind Clinical Trial of a Novel Formulation of 5% Minoxidil Topical Foam Versus Placebo in the Treatment of Androgenetic Alopecia in Men," *Journal of the American Academy of Dermatology* 57, no. 5 (November 2007): 767–74; Richard A. Preston et al., "Placebo-Associated Blood Pressure Response and Adverse Effects in the Treatment of Hypertension: Observations from a Department of Veterans Affairs Cooperative Study," *Archives of Internal Medicine* 160, no. 10 (May 22, 2000): 1449–54; H. V. Allington, "Review of the Psychotherapy of Warts," *AMA Archives of Dermatology and Syphilology* 66, no. 3 (1952): 316–26; H. Vollmer, "Treatment of Warts by Suggestion," *Psychosomatic Medicine* 8 (March 1946): 138–42; Montague Ullman and Stephanie Dudek, "On the Psyche and Warts: Hypnotic Suggestion and Warts," *Psychosomatic Medicine* 22, no. 1 (January 1, 1960): 437–88; Anton J. M. De Craen et al., "Placebo Effect in the Treatment of Duodenal Ulcer," *British Journal of Clinical Pharmacology* 48, no. 6 (December 1999): 853–60; F. K. Abbot, M. Mack, and S. Wolf, "The Action of Banthine on the Stomach and Duodenum of Man with Observations on the Effects of Placebos," *Gastroenterology* 20, no. 2 (February 1952): 249–61; Talbot, "The Placebo Prescription"; Paul L. Canner, Sandra A. Forman, and Gerard J. Prud'homme, "Influence of Adherence to Treatment and Response of Cholesterol on Mortality in the Coronary Drug Project," *New England Journal of Medicine* 303 (October 30, 1980): 1038–41; Ibrahim Hashish et al., "Reduction of Postoperative Pain and Swelling by Ultrasound Treatment: A Placebo Effect," *Pain* 33, no. 3 (June 1988): 303–11; Raúl de la Fuente-Fernández et al., "Expectation and Dopamine Release: Mechanism of the Placebo Effect in Parkinson's Disease," *Science* 293, no. 5532 (August 10, 2001): 1164–66; C. Kirschbaum et al., "Conditioning of Drug-Induced Immunomodulation in Human Volunteers: A European Collaborative Study," *British Journal of Clinical Psychology* 31, no. 4 (November 1992): 459–72; Predrag Petrovic et al., "Placebo and Opioid Analgesia: Imaging a Shared Neuronal Network," *Science* 295, no. 5560 (March 1, 2002): 1737–40; Matthew D. Lieberman et al., "The Neural Correlates of Placebo Effects: A Disruption Account," *Neuroimage* 22, no. 1 (May 2004): 447–55; Tor D. Wager et al., "Placebo-Induced Changes in fMRI in the Anticipation and Experience of Pain," *Science* 303, no. 5661 (February 20, 2004): 1162–67.

15. Irving Kirsch, "Response Expectancy as a Determinant of Experience and Behavior," *American Psychologist* 40, no. 11 (November 1985): 1189–1202.

16. I. Wickramasekera, "A Conditioned Response Model of the Placebo Effect: Predictions from the Model," *Biofeedback and Self-Regulation* 5, no. 1 (March 1980): 5–18; Nicholas J. Voudouris, Connie L. Peck, and Grahame Coleman, "Conditioned Response Models of Placebo Phenomena: Further Support," *Pain* 38, no. 1 (July 1989): 109–16.

17. Asbjørn Hróbjartsson and Peter C. Gøtzsche, "Is the Placebo Powerless? An Analysis of Clinical Trials Comparing Placebo with No Treatment," *New England Journal of Medicine* 344, no. 21 (May 24, 2001): 1594–1602.

18. Daniel E. Moerman and Wayne B. Jonas, "Deconstructing the Placebo Effect and Finding the Meaning Response," *Annals of Internal Medicine* 136, no. 6 (March 19, 2002): 471–76.

19. Fabrizio Benedetti, *Placebo Effects: Understanding the Mechanisms in Health and Disease* (New York: Oxford University Press, 2009): 29.

20. Jon D. Levine, Newton C. Gordon, and Howard L. Fields, "The Mechanism of Placebo Analgesia," *Lancet* 312, no. 8091 (September 23, 1978): 654–57.

21. R. Ader and N. Cohen, "Behaviorally Conditioned Immunosuppression," *Psychosomatic Medicine* 37, no. 4 (July/August 1975): 333–40.

22. Evans, *Placebo: Mind over Matter in Modern Medicine*, 44–69.

23. Benedetti et al., "Loss of Expectation-Related Mechanisms in Alzheimer's Disease Makes Analgesic Therapies Less Effective."

24. David J. Scott et al., "Individual Differences in Reward Responding Explain Placebo-Induced Expectations and Effects," *Neuron* 55, no. 2 (July 19, 2007): 325–36.

25. Caryle Hirshberg and Brendan O'Regan, *Spontaneous Remission: An Annotated Bibliography* (Petaluma, CA: Institute of Noetic Sciences, 1993), http://noetic.org/library /publication-books/spontaneous-remission-annotated-bibliography/.

26. Ibid.

Chapter 2

1. D. P. Phillips, T. E. Ruth, and L. M. Wagner, "Psychology and Survival," *Lancet* 342, no. 8880 (November 6, 1993): 1142–45.

2. S. M. Woods, J. Natterson, and J. Silverman, "Medical Students' Disease: Hypochondriasis in Medical Education," *Journal of Medical Education* 41, no. 8 (August 1966): 785–90.

3. Bernie S. Siegel, *Love, Medicine & Miracles* (New York: Harper & Row, 1986), 133.

4. Pierre Kissel and Dominique Barrucand, *Placebos et Effet Placebo en Médecine* (Paris: Masson, 1964).

5. Stanley Schachter and Jerome Singer, "Cognitive, Social and Physiological Determinants of Emotional State," *Psychological Review* 69, no. 5 (September 1962): 379–99.

6. Norman Cousins, *Anatomy of an Illness: As Perceived by the Patient* (New York: W. W. Norton & Company, 1979), 59.

7. Samuel F. Dworkin et al., "Cognitive Reversal of Expected Nitrous Oxide Analgesia for Acute Pain," *Anesthesia and Analgesia* 62, no. 12 (December 1983): 1073–77.

8. Avraham Schweiger and Allen Parducci, "Nocebo: The Psychologic Induction of Pain," *Pavlovian Journal of Biological Science* 16, no. 3 (July–September 1981): 140–43.

9. Brian Reid, "The Nocebo Effect: The Placebo Effect's Evil Twin," *Washington Post*, April 30, 2002.

10. Ibid.

11. Anthony Robbins, *Unlimited Power: The New Science of Personal Achievement* (New York: Free Press, 1986).

12. Bennett G. Braun, ed., *The Treatment of Multiple Personality Disorder* (Arlington, VA: American Psychiatric Press, 1986).

13. Richard L. Kradin, *The Placebo Response and the Power of Unconscious Healing* (New York: Routledge, 2008), 151.

14. Martina Amanzio et al., "A Systematic Review of Adverse Events in Placebo Groups of Anti-migraine Clinical Trials," *Pain* 146, no. 3 (December 5, 2009): 261–69.

15. Walter B. Cannon, "Voodoo Death," *American Anthropologist* 44, no. 2 (April–June, 1942): 169–81.

16. John Cloud, "The Flip Side of Placebos: The Nocebo Effect," *Time*, October 13, 2009, http://www.time.com/time/magazine/article/0,9171,1931727,00.html.

17. Sanford I. Cohen, "Voodoo Death, the Stress Response, and AIDS," *Advanced Biochemical Psychopharmacology* 44 (1998): 95–109.

18. D. N. Ruble, "Premenstrual Symptoms: A Reinterpretation," *Science* 197, no. 4300 (July 15, 1977): 291–292.

19. Michael J. Colligan and Lawrence R. Murphy, "Mass Psychogenic Illness in Organizations: An Overview," *Journal of Occupational Psychology* 52, no. 2 (June 1979): 77–90.

20. Fabrizio Benedetti et al., "The Biochemical and Neuroendocrine Bases of the Hyperalgesic Nocebo Effect," *Journal of Neuroscience* 26, no. 46 (November 15, 2006): 12014–22.

21. Bruce Lipton, *The Biology of Belief: Unleashing the Power of Consciousness, Matter and Miracles* (Carlsbad, CA: Hay House, 2008).

22. Robert A. Waterland and Randy L. Jirtle, "Transposable Elements: Targets for Early Nutritional Effects on Epigenetic Gene Regulation," *Molecular and Cellular Biology* 23, no. 15 (August 2003): 5293–5300; Eva Jablonka and Marion J. Lamb, *Epigenetic Inheritance and Evolution: The Lamarckian Dimension* (Oxford: Oxford University Press, 1995).

23. Walter C. Willett, "Balancing Life-Style and Genomics Research for Disease Prevention," *Science* 296, no. 5568 (April 26, 2002): 695–98.

24. Peter D. Gluckman and Mark A. Hanson, "Living with the Past: Evolution, Development, and Patterns of Disease," *Science* 305, no. 5691 (September 17, 2004): 1733–36.

25. Peter W. Nathanielsz, *Life in the Womb: The Origin of Health and Disease* (New York: Promethean Press, 1999).

26. James W. Prescott, Scientific Director, *Rock A Bye Baby* (New York: Time-Life Films, 1970).

27. Patrick Bateson et al., "Developmental Plasticity and Human Health," *Nature* 430, no. 6998 (July 22, 2004): 419–21.

Chapter 3

1. "One Scholar's Take on the Power of the Placebo," *Science Friday,* NPR, January 6, 2012, http://m.npr.org/news/Health/144794035.

2. Michael Specter, "The Power of Nothing," *New Yorker,* December 12, 2011.

3. Michael E. Wechsler et al., "Active Albuterol or Placebo, Sham Acupuncture, or No Intervention in Asthma," *New England Journal of Medicine* 365 (July 14, 2011): 119–26.

4. Lawrence D. Egbert et al., "Reduction of Postoperative Pain by Encouragement and Instruction of Patients: A Study of Doctor-Patient Rapport," *New England Journal of Medicine* 270 (April 16, 1964): 825–27.

5. Ibid.

6. K. B. Thomas, "General Practice Consultations: Is There Any Point in Being Positive?" *British Medical Journal* 294, no. 6581 (May 9, 1987): 1200–1202.

7. Fabrizio Benedetti et al., "When Words Are Painful: Unraveling the Mechanisms of the Nocebo Effect," *Neuroscience* 147, no. 2 (June 29, 2007): 260–71.

8. Richard H. Gracely et al., "Clinicians' Expectations Influence Placebo Analgesia," *Lancet* 325, no. 8419 (January 5, 1985): 43.

9. Janice L. Krupnick et al., "The Role of the Therapeutic Alliance in Psychotherapy and Pharmacotherapy Outcome: Findings in the National Institute of Mental Health Treatment of Depression Collaborative Research Program," *Journal of Consulting and Clinical Psychology* 64, no. 3 (June 1996): 532–39.

10. Ted J. Kaptchuk et al., "Components of Placebo Effect: Randomised Controlled Trial in Patients with Irritable Bowel Syndrome," *British Medical Journal* 336, no. 7651 (May 1, 2008): 999–1003.

11. A. H. Sinclair-Gieben and D. Chalmers, "Evaluation of Treatment of Warts by Hypnosis," *Lancet* 274, no. 7101 (October 3, 1959): 480–82; Owen S. Surman, Sheldon K. Gottlieb, and Thomas P. Hackett, "Hypnotic Treatment of a Child with Warts," *American Journal of Clinical Hypnosis* 15, no. 1 (July 1972): 12–14.

12. Curtis E. Margo, "The Placebo Effect," *Survey of Ophthalmology* 44, no. 1 (July/August

1999): 33–34; Nicholas J. Voudouris, Connie L. Peck, and Grahame Coleman, "Conditioned Response Models of Placebo Phenomena: Further Support," *Pain* 38, no. 1 (July 1989): 109–16; Steve Stewart-Williams and John Podd, "The Placebo Effect: Dissolving the Expectancy Versus Conditioning Debate," *Psychology Bulletin* 130, no. 2 (March 2004): 324–40.

13. Desonta Holder, "Health: Beware Negative Self-Fulfilling Prophecy," *Seattle Times,* January 2, 2008, http://seattletimes.nwsource.com/html/health/2004101546 _fearofdying02.html.

14. Julia Kleinhenz et al., "Randomised Clinical Trial Comparing the Effects of Acupuncture and a Newly Designed Placebo Needle in Rotator Cuff Tendinitis," *Pain* 83, no. 2 (November 1, 1999): 235–41; J. Vas et al., "Acupuncture as a Complementary Therapy to the Pharmacological Treatment of Osteoarthritis of the Knee: Randomised Controlled Trial," *British Medical Journal* 329, no. 7476 (November 20, 2004): 1216–19; Juan Antonio Guerra de Hoyos et al., "Randomised Trial of Long-Term Effect of Acupuncture for Shoulder Pain," *Pain* 112, no. 3 (December 2004): 289–98.

15. Edzard Ernst and Adrian R. White, "Acupuncture for Back Pain: A Meta-Analysis of Randomized Controlled Trials," *Archives of Internal Medicine* 158, no. 20 (November 9, 1998): 2235–41; Matthias Karst et al., "Pressure Pain Threshold and Needle Acupuncture in Chronic Tension-Type Headache: A Double-Blind Placebo-Controlled Study," *Pain* 88, no. 2 (November 2000): 199–203; Matthias Karst et al., "Needle Acupuncture in Tension-Type Headache: A Randomized, Placebo-Controlled Study," *Cephalalgia* 21, no. 6 (July 2001): 637–42; Matthias Karst et al., "Acupuncture in the Treatment of Alcohol Withdrawal Symptoms: A Randomized, Placebo-Controlled Inpatient Study," *Addiction Biology* 7, no. 4 (October 2002): 415–19; Jongbae Park et al., "Acupuncture for Subacute Stroke Rehabilitation: A Sham-Controlled, Subject-and Assessor-Blind, Randomized Trial," *Archives of Internal Medicine* 165, no. 17 (September 26, 2005): 2026–31; K. Streitberger et al., "Effect of Acupuncture Compared with Placebo-Acupuncture at P6 as Additional Antiemetic Prophylaxis in High-Dose Chemotherapy and Autologous Peripheral Blood Stem Cell Transplantation: A Randomized Controlled Single-Blind Trial," *Clinical Cancer Research* 9, no. 7 (July 2003): 2538–44; K. Streitberger et al., "Acupuncture Compared to Placebo-Acupuncture for Postoperative Nausea and Vomiting Prophylaxis: A Randomised Placebo-Controlled Patient and Observer Blind Trial," *Anaesthesia* 59, no. 2 (February 2004): 142–49; Matthias Fink et al., "Needle Acupuncture in Chronic Poststroke Leg Spasticity," *Archives of Physical Medicine and Rehabilitation* 85, no. 4 (April 2004): 667–72; M. Linde et al., "Role of the Needling Per Se in Acupuncture as Prophylaxis for Menstrually Related Migraine: A Randomized Placebo-Controlled Study," *Cephalalgia* 25, no. 1 (January 2005): 41–47.

16. Anita Catlin and Rebecca L. Taylor-Ford, "Investigation of Standard Care Versus Sham Reiki Placebo Versus Actual Reiki Therapy to Enhance Comfort and Well-Being in a Chemotherapy Infusion Center," *Oncology Nursing Forum* 38, no. 3 (May 2011): E212–E220.

17. J. Kleijnen, P. Knipschild, and G. ter Riet, "Clinical Trials of Homoeopathy," *British Medical Journal* 302, no. 6772 (February 9, 1991): 316–23.

18. Aijing Shang et al., "Are the Clinical Effects of Homoeopathy Placebo Effects? Com-

parative Study of Placebo-Controlled Trials of Homoeopathy and Allopathy," *Lancet* 366, no. 9487 (August 27–September 2, 2005): 726–32.

19. "The End of Homeopathy," editorial, *Lancet* 366, no. 9487 (August 27–September 2, 2005): 690.

20. Iris R. Bell, "All Evidence Is Equal, but Some Evidence Is More Equal than Others: Can Logic Prevail over Emotion in the Homeopathy Debate?" *Journal of Alternative and Complementary Medicine* 11, no. 5 (October 2005): 763–69.

21. David Spiegel and Anne Harrington, "What Is the Placebo Worth?" *British Medical Journal* 336, no. 7651 (May 3, 2008): 967–68.

22. Mary L. Smith and Gene V. Glass, "Meta-Analysis of Psychotherapy Outcome Studies," *American Psychologist* 32, no. 9 (September 1977): 752–60.

23. Hans H. Strupp and Suzanne W. Hadley, "Specific vs. Nonspecific Factors in Psychotherapy: A Controlled Study of Outcome," *Archives of General Psychiatry* 36, no. 10 (September 1979): 1125–36.

24. Arthur Kleinman, *Rethinking Psychiatry: From Cultural Category to Personal Experience* (New York: Free Press, 1991).

25. Ted J. Kaptchuk et al., "Complementary Medicine: Efficacy Beyond the Placebo Effect," in *Complementary Medicine: An Objective Appraisal*, ed. Edzard Ernst (Oxford: Butterworth-Heinemann, 1996), 42–70.

26. Michael Talbot, *The Holographic Universe* (New York: HarperCollins, 1991), 107.

Chapter 4

1. Richard A. Dienstbier, "Arousal and Physiological Toughness: Implications for Mental and Physical Health," *Psychological Review* 96, no. 1 (January 1989): 84–100; Marianne Frankenhaeuser, "The Psychophysiology of Workload, Stress, and Health: Comparison Between the Sexes," *Annals of Behavioral Medicine* 13, no. 4 (1991): 197–204; Shelley E. Taylor, *Health Psychology* (New York: McGraw-Hill, 1999), 168–201.

Chapter 5

1. Malcolm Gladwell, *Outliers: The Story of Success* (New York: Little, Brown & Company, 2008), 7.

2. J. S. House, K. R. Landis, and D. Umberson, "Social Relationships and Health," *Science* 241, no. 4865 (July 29, 1988): 540–45.

3. Ron Grossman and Charles Leroux, "A New 'Roseto Effect': 'People Are Nourished by Other People,'" *Chicago Tribune*, October 11, 1996, http://articles.chicagotribune.com/1996-10-11/news/9610110254_1_satellite-dishes-outsiders-town/2.

4. Lisa F. Berkman and S. Leonard Syme, "Social Networks, Host Resistance, and Mortality: A Nine-Year Follow-Up Study of Alameda County Residents," *American Journal of Epidemiology* 109, no. 2 (February 1, 1979): 186–204.

5. Peggy Reynolds and George A. Kaplan, "Social Connections and Risk for Cancer: Prospective Evidence from the Alameda County Study," *Behavioral Medicine* 16, no. 3 (Fall 1990): 101–10.

6. Thomas A. Glass et al., "Population Based Study of Social and Productive Activities as Predictors of Survival among Elderly Americans," *British Medical Journal* 319 (August 21, 1999): 478.

7. L. C. Giles et al., "Effect of Social Networks on 10 Year Survival in Very Old Australians: The Australian Longitudinal Study of Aging," *Journal of Epidemiological Community Health* 59, no. 7 (July 2005): 574–79; J. S. House, C. Robbins, and H. L. Metzner, "The Association of Social Relationships and Activities with Mortality: Prospective Evidence from the Tecumseh Community Health Study," *American Journal of Epidemiology* 116, no. 1 (July 1982): 123–40.

8. Candyce H. Kroenke et al., "Social Networks, Social Support, and Survival after Breast Cancer Diagnosis," *Journal of Clinical Oncology* 24, no. 7 (March 1, 2006): 1105–11.

9. Annika Rosengren, Lars Wilhelmsen, and Kristina Orth-Gomér, "Coronary Disease in Relation to Social Support and Social Class in Swedish Men: A 15 Year Follow-Up in the Study of Men Born in 1933," *European Heart Journal* 25, no. 1 (January 2004): 56–63.

10. Jo Marchant, "Heal Thyself: Trust People," *NewScientist,* August 30, 2011, http://www.newscientist.com/article/mg21128271.800-heal-thyself-trust-people.html.

11. W. J. Strawbridge et al., "Frequent Attendance at Religious Services and Mortality over 28 Years," *American Journal of Public Health* 87, no. 6 (June 1997): 957–61.

12. D. Oman and D. Reed, "Religion and Mortality among the Community-Dwelling Elderly," *American Journal of Public Health* 88, no. 10 (October 1998): 1469–75.

13. T. E. Oxman, D. H. Freeman, and E. D. Manheimer, "Lack of Social Participation or Religious Strength and Comfort as Risk Factors for Death after Cardiac Surgery in the Elderly," *Psychosomatic Medicine* 57, no. 1 (January/February 1995): 5–15.

14. Harold G. Koenig et al., "Modeling the Cross-Sectional Relationships Between Religion, Physical Health, Social Support, and Depressive Symptoms," *American Journal of Geriatric Psychology* 5, no. 2 (Spring 1997): 131–44.

15. Christopher G. Ellison and Jeffrey S. Levin, "The Religion-Health Connection: Evidence, Theory, and Future Directions," *Health Education and Behavior* 25, no. 6 (December 1998): 700–720.

16. Robert A. Hummer et al., "Religious Involvement and U.S. Adult Mortality," *Demography* 36, no. 2 (May 1999): 273–85; Michael E. McCullough et al., "Religious Involvement and Mortality: A Meta-Analytic Review," *Health Psychology* 19, no. 3 (May 2000): 211–22.

17. Patrick R. Steffen et al., "Religious Coping, Ethnicity, and Ambulatory Blood Pressure," *Psychosomatic Medicine* 63, no. 4 (July–August 2001): 523–30; John Gartner, Dave B. Larson, and George D. Allen, "Religious Commitment and Mental Health: A Review of the Empirical Literature," *Journal of Psychology and Theology* 19, no. 1 (Spring 1991): 6–25; Harold G. Koenig and David B. Larson, "Religion and Mental Health: Evidence for an Association," *International Review of Psychiatry* 13, no. 2

(2001): 67–78; Sandra E. Sephton et al., "Spiritual Expression and Immune Status in Women with Metastatic Breast Cancer: An Exploratory Study," *Breast Journal* 7, no. 5 (September/October 2001): 345–53; Teresa E. Woods et al., "Religiosity Is Associated with Affective and Immune Status in Symptomatic HIV-Infected Gay Men," *Journal of Psychosomatic Research* 46, no. 2 (February 1999): 165–76.

18. Joseph L. Lyon, Kent Gardner, and Richard E. Gress, "Cancer Incidence in Mormons and Non-Mormons in Utah (United States) 1971–1985," *Cancer Causes & Control* 5, no. 2 (March 1994): 149–56.

19. William J. Strawbridge, Richard D. Cohen, and Sarah J. Shema, "Comparative Strength of Association between Religious Attendance and Survival," *International Journal of Psychiatry in Medicine* 30, no. 4 (2000): 299–308; Doug Oman et al., "Religious Attendance and Cause of Death Over 31 Years," *International Journal of Psychiatry in Medicine* 32, no. 1 (2002): 69–89.

20. Daniel N. McIntosh, Roxane Cohen Silver, and Camille B. Wortman, "Religion's Role in Adjustment to a Negative Life Event: Coping with the Loss of a Child," *Journal of Personality and Social Psychology* 65, no. 4 (October 1993): 812–21.

21. Michael E. McCullough and Everett L. Worthington, Jr., "Religion and the Forgiving Personality," *Journal of Personality* 67, no. 6 (December 1999): 1141–64.

22. Melvin Pollner, "Divine Relations, Social Relations, and Well-Being," *Journal of Health and Social Behavior* 30 no. 1 (March 1989): 92–104.

23. Kenneth I. Pargament, "The Psychology of Religion *and* Spirituality?: Yes and No," *International Journal for the Psychology of Religion* 9, no. 1 (1999): 3–16.

24. Harold G. Koenig, Kenneth I. Pargament, and Julie Nielsen, "Religious Coping and Health Status in Medically Ill Hospitalized Older Adults," *Journal of Nervous and Mental Disease* 186, no. 9 (September 1998): 513–21.

25. Pamela Kotler and Deborah Lee Wingard, "The Effect of Occupational, Marital and Parental Roles on Mortality: The Alameda County Study," *American Journal of Public Health* 79, no. 5 (May 1989): 607–12.

26. Robert M. Kaplan and Richard G. Kronick, "Marital Status and Longevity in the United States Population," *Journal of Epidemiology and Community Health* 60, no. 9 (September 2006): 760–65.

27. Brigham Young University, "Happily Marrieds Have Lower Blood Pressure than Social Singles," *ScienceDaily*, March 21, 2008, http://www.sciencedaily.com/releases/2008/03/080320192610.htm.

28. American Academy of Sleep Medicine, "More Marital Happiness = Less Sleep Complaints," *ScienceDaily*, June 11, 2008, http://www.sciencedaily.com/releases/2008/06/080609071336.htm.

29. Sheree J. Gibb, David M. Fergusson, and L. John Horwood, "Relationship Duration and Mental Health Outcomes: Findings from a 30-Year Longitudinal Study," *British Journal of Psychiatry* 198, no. 1 (2011): 24–30.

30. Dario Maestripieri et al., "Between- and Within-Sex Variation in Hormonal Responses to Psychological Stress in a Large Sample of College Students," *Stress* 13, no. 5 (September 2010): 413–24; "Relationships Are Good for Your Health: Being Married

or in a Long-Term Relationship Improves Your Ability to Deal with Stress, a New Study Suggests," *Telegraph*, August 18, 2010, http://www.telegraph.co.uk/health /healthnews/7952466/Relationships-are-good-for-your-health.html.

31. BMJ–British Medical Journal, "Marriage Is Good for Physical and Mental Health, Study Finds," *ScienceDaily*, January 28, 2011, http://www.sciencedaily.com /releases/2011/01/110127205853.htm.

32. Ohio State University, "Marital Problems Lead to Poorer Outcomes for Breast Cancer Patients," *ScienceDaily*, December 10, 2008, http://www.sciencedaily.com /releases/2008/12/081208123304.htm.

33. Wiley-Blackwell, "Intimate Abuse Study Finds Clear Links with Poor Health and Calls for Holistic Primary Care Approach," *ScienceDaily*, July 6, 2009, http://www .sciencedaily.com/releases/2009/07/090706090438.htm.

34. James W. Pennebaker and Robin C. O'Heeron, "Confiding in Others and Illness Rate among Spouses of Suicide and Accidental-Death Victims," *Journal of Abnormal Psychology* 93, no. 4 (November 1984): 473–76.

35. George Davey Smith, Stephen Frankel, and John Yarnell, "Sex and Death: Are They Related? Findings from the Caerphilly Cohort Study," *British Medical Journal* 315, no. 7133 (December 20–27, 1997): 1641–44; Erdman B. Palmore, "Predictors of the Longevity Difference: A 25-Year Follow-Up," *Gerontologist* 22, no. 6 (December 1982): 513–18; G. Persson, "Five-Year Mortality in a 70-Year-Old Urban Population in Relation to Psychiatric Diagnosis, Personality, Sexuality and Early Parental Death," *Acta Psychiatrica Scandinavica* 64, no. 3 (September 1981): 244–53; S. Ebrahim et al., "Sexual Intercourse and Risk of Ischaemic Stroke and Coronary Heart Disease: The Caerphilly Study," *Journal of Epidemiology and Community Health* 56, no. 2 (February 2002): 99–102; Monique G. Lê, Annie Bacheloti, and Catherine Hill, "Characteristics of Reproductive Life and Risk of Breast Cancer in a Case-Control Study of Young Nulliparous Women," *Journal of Clinical Epidemiology* 42, no. 12 (1989): 1227–33; Carl J. Charnetski and Francis X. Brennan, *Feeling Good Is Good for You: How Pleasure Can Boost Your Immune System and Lengthen Your Life* (Emmaus, PA: Rodale Books, 2001); Carol Rinkleib Ellison, *Women's Sexualities* (Oakland, CA: New Harbinger Publications, Inc., 2000); David Weeks and Jamie James, *Secrets of the Superyoung* (New York: Berkley Books, 1999); Winnifred B. Cutler, *Love Cycles: The Science of Intimacy* (New York: Villard Books, 1991); Helen Singer Kaplan, "Desire? Why and How It Changes," *Redbook*, October 1984, as cited in B. R. Komisaruk and B. Whipple, "The Suppression of Pain by Genital Stimulation in Females," *Annual Review of Sex Research* 6 (1995): 151–86; D. Shapiro, "Effect of Chronic Low Back Pain on Sexuality," *Medical Aspects of Human Sexuality* 17 (1983): 241–45, as cited in Komisaruk and Whipple, "The Suppression of Pain by Genital Stimulation in Females"; Beverly Whipple and Barry R. Komisaruk, "Elevation of Pain Threshold by Vaginal Stimulation in Women," *Pain* 21, no. 4 (April 1985): 357–67; Randolph W. Evans and James R. Couch, "Orgasm and Migraine," *Headache* 41, no. 5 (May 2001): 512–14; Joseph A. Catania and Charles B. White, "Sexuality in an Aged Sample: Cognitive Determinants of Masturbation," *Archives of Sexual Behavior* 11, no. 3 (June 1982): 237–45; David J. Weeks, "Sex for the Mature Adult: Health, Self-Esteem and Countering Ageist Stereotypes," *Sexual and Relationship Therapy* 17, no. 3 (2002): 231–40; Pamela Warner and John Bancroft, "Mood, Sexuality, Oral Contraceptives and the Menstru-

al Cycle," *Journal of Psychosomatic Research* 32, no. 4–5 (1988): 417–27; Edward O. Laumann et al., *The Social Organization of Sexuality: Sexual Practice in the United States* (Chicago: University of Chicago, 1994).

36. Vello Sermat, "Some Situational and Personality Correlates of Loneliness," in *The Anatomy of Loneliness*, ed. Joseph Hartog, J. Ralph Audy, and Yehudi A. Cohen (New York: International Universities Press, 1980).

37. C. M. Rubenstein and P. Shaver, "Loneliness in Two Northeastern Cities."

38. Roelof Hortulanus, Anja Machielse, and Ludwien Meeuwesen, *Social Isolation in Modern Society* (New York: Routledge, 2004).

39. Robert D. Putnam, *Bowling Alone: The Collapse and Revival of American Community* (New York: Simon & Schuster, 2001).

40. John T. Cacioppo et al., "Loneliness and Health: Potential Mechanisms," *Psychosomatic Medicine* 64, no. 3 (May/June 2002): 407–17.

41. Andrew Steptoe et al., "Loneliness and Neuroendocrine, Cardiovascular, and Inflammatory Stress Responses in Middle-Aged Men and Women," *Psychoneuroendocrinology* 29, no. 5 (June 2004): 593–611.

42. Dara Sorkin, Karen S. Rook, and John L. Lu, "Loneliness, Lack of Emotional Support, Lack of Companionship, and the Likelihood of Having a Heart Condition in an Elderly Sample," *Annals of Behavioral Medicine* 24, no. 4 (Fall 2002): 290–98; Cyndy M. Fox et al., "Loneliness, Emotional Repression, Marital Quality, and Major Life Events in Women Who Develop Breast Cancer," *Journal of Community Health* 19, no. 6 (December 1994): 467–82; Robert S. Wilson et al., "Loneliness and Risk of Alzheimer Disease," *Archives of General Psychiatry* 64, no. 2 (February 2007): 234–40; Ariel Stravynski and Richard Boyer, "Loneliness in Relation to Suicide Ideation and Parasuicide: A Population-Wide Study," *Suicide and Life-Threatening Behavior* 31, no. 1 (Spring 2001): 32–40.

43. J. Herlitz et al., "The Feeling of Loneliness prior to Coronary Artery Bypass Grafting Might Be a Predictor of Short- and Long-Term Postoperative Mortality," *European Journal of Vascular and Endovascular Surgery* 16, no. 2 (August 1998): 120–25.

44. Cacioppo et al., "Loneliness and Health: Potential Mechanisms."

45. John T. Cacioppo et al., "Lonely Traits and Concomitant Physiological Processes: The MacArthur Social Neuroscience Studies," *International Journal of Psychophysiology* 35, no. 2–3 (March 2000): 143–54.

46. Janice K. Kiecolt-Glaser et al., "Psychosocial Modifiers of Immunocompetence in Medical Students," *Psychosomatic Medicine* 46, no. 1 (January/February 1984): 7–14; Janice K. Kiecolt-Glaser et al., "Urinary Cortisol Levels, Cellular Immunocompetency, and Loneliness in Psychiatric Patients," *Psychosomatic Medicine* 46, no. 1 (January/February 1984): 15–23; Sarah D. Pressman et al., "Loneliness, Social Network Size, and Immune Response to Influenza Vaccination in College Freshmen," *Health Psychology* 24, no. 3 (May 2005): 297–306; Bert N. Uchino, John T. Cacioppo, and Janice K. Kiecolt-Glaser, "The Relationship between Support and Physiological Processes: A Review with Emphasis on Underlying Mechanisms and Implications for Health," *Psychological Bulletin* 119, no. 3 (May 1996): 488–531.

47. James J. Lynch, *The Broken Heart* (New York: Basic Books, 1977), 84.

48. Karen S. Rook, "The Negative Side of Social Interaction: Impact on Psychological Well-Being," *Journal of Personality and Social Psychology* 46, no. 5 (May 1984): 1097–1108.

49. Brené Brown, *The Gifts of Imperfection* (Center City, MN: Hazelden, 2010).

Chapter 6

1. K. Morioka, "Work Till You Drop," *New Labor Forum* 13, no. 1 (Spring 2004): 81–85.

2. Becky Barrow, "Stress 'Is Top Cause of Workplace Sickness' and Is So Widespread It's Dubbed the 'Black Death of the 21st Century,'" *MailOnline*, October 5, 2011, http://www.dailymail.co.uk/health/article-2045309/Stress-Top-cause-workplace-sickness-dubbed-Black-Death-21st-century.html.

3. Katsuo Nishiyama and Jeffrey V. Johnson, "Karoshi—Death from Overwork: Occupational Health Consequences of Japanese Production Management," *International Journal of Health Services* 27, no. 4 (1997), 627–41.

4. Morioka, "Work Till You Drop."

5. Ronald E. Yates, "Japanese Live . . . and Die . . . for Their Work," *Chicago Tribune*, November 13, 1988, http://articles.chicagotribune.com/1988-11-13/news/8802150740_1_karoshi-japanese-health-and-welfare.

6. Matthew Reiss, "American Karoshi," *New Internationalist* 343 (March 2002).

7. Alina Tugend, "Want to Work Better? Take a Vacation," *New York Times*, June 9, 2008, http://www.nytimes.com/2008/06/09/business/worldbusiness/09iht-vac.4.13584260.html?_r=2.

8. Brooks B. Gump and Karen A. Matthews, "Are Vacations Good for Your Health? The 9-Year Mortality Experience after the Multiple Risk Factor Intervention Trial," *Psychosomatic Medicine* 62, no. 5 (September/October 2000): 608–12.

9. Elaine D. Eaker, Joan Pinsky, and William P. Castelli, "Myocardial Infarction and Coronary Death among Women: Psychosocial Predictors from a 20-Year Follow-Up of Women in the Framingham Study," *American Journal of Epidemiology* 135, no. 8 (April 15, 1992): 854–64.

10. S. L. Manne and A. J. Zautra, "Spouse Criticism and Support: Their Association with Coping and Psychological Adjustment among Women with Rheumatoid Arthritis," *Journal of Personality and Social Psychology* 56, no. 4 (April 1989): 608–17; Mary C. Davis, Alex J. Zautra, and John W. Reich, "Vulnerability to Stress among Women in Chronic Pain from Fibromyalgia and Osteoarthritis," *Annals of Behavioral Medicine* 23, no. 3 (Summer 2001): 215–26; A. J. Zautra, L. M. Johnson, and M. C. Davis, "Positive Affect as a Source of Resilience for Women in Chronic Pain," *Journal of Consulting and Clinical Psychology* 73, no. 2 (April 2005): 212–20.

11. B. A. Huyser and J. C. Parker, "Negative Affect and Pain in Arthritis," *Rheumatic Disease Clinics of North America* 25, no. 1 (February 1999): 105–21; S. A. McLean et

al., "Momentary Relationship between Cortisol Secretion and Symptoms in Patients with Fibromyalgia," *Arthritis and Rheumatism* 52, no. 11 (November 2005): 3660–69; S. A. McLean et al., "Cerebrospinal Fluid Corticotropin-Releasing Factor Concentration Is Associated with Pain but Not Fatigue Symptoms in Patients with Fibromyalgia," *Neuropsychopharmacology* 31, no. 12 (December 2006), 2776–82.

12. L. Bendtsen, "Central and Peripheral Sensitization in Tension-Type Headache," *Current Pain Headache Reports* 7, no. 6 (December 2003): 460–65.

13. Ashley E. Nixon et al., "Can Work Make You Sick? A Meta-Analysis of the Relationships between Job Stressors and Physical Symptoms," *Work & Stress* 25, no. 1 (January–March 2011): 1–22; S. T. Gura, "Yoga for Stress Reduction and Injury Prevention at Work," *Work: Journal of Prevention, Assessment and Rehabilitation* 19, no. 1 (2002): 3–7.

14. R. Rau et al., "Psychosocial Work Characteristics and Perceived Control in Relation to Cardiovascular Rewind at Night," *Journal of Occupational Health Psychology* 6, no. 3 (July 2001): 171–81; K. A. Ertel, K. Karestan, and L. F. Berkman, "Incorporating Home Demands into Models of Job Strain: Findings from the Work, Family, and Health Network," *Journal of Occupational and Environmental Medicine* 50, no. 11 (November 2008): 1244–52; T. Roth and S. Ancoli-Israel, "Daytime Consequences and Correlates of Insomnia in the United States: Results of the 1991 National Sleep Foundation Survey. II," *Sleep* 22, no. 2 (May 1, 1999): 354–58; M. Jansson and S. J. Linton, "Psychosocial Work Stressors in the Development and Maintenance of Insomnia: A Prospective Study," *Journal of Occupational Health Psychology* 11, no. 3 (July 2006): 241–48.

15. Steven J. Linton and Ing-Liss Bryngelsson, "Insomnia and Its Relationship to Work and Health in a Working-Age Population," *Journal of Occupational Rehabilitation* 10, no. 2 (June 2000): 169–83.

16. G. Aguilera, "Regulation of Pituitary ACTH Secretion during Chronic Stress," *Frontiers in Neuroendocrinology* 15, no. 4 (December 1994): 321–50.

17. A. J. Dittner, S. C. Wessely, and R. G. Brown, "The Assessment of Fatigue: A Practical Guide for Clinicians and Researchers," *Journal of Psychosomatic Research* 56, no. 2 (February 2004): 157–70; Pascal M. L. Franssen et al., "The Association between Chronic Diseases and Fatigue in the Working Population," *Journal of Psychosomatic Research* 54, no. 4 (April 2003): 339–44.

18. Mark A. Demitrack et al., "Evidence for Impaired Activation of the Hypothalamic-Pituitary-Adrenal Axis in Patients with Chronic Fatigue Syndrome," *Journal of Clinical Endocrinology and Metabolism* 73, no. 6 (December 1991): 1224–34.

19. A. K. Smith et al., "Polymorphisms in Genes Regulating the HPA Axis Associated with Empirically Delineated Classes of Unexplained Chronic Fatigue," *Pharmacogenomics* 7, no. 3 (April 2006): 387–94.

20. Jack Sparacino, "Blood Pressure, Stress and Mental Health," *Nursing Research* 31, no. 2 (March–April 1982): 89–94.

21. Nixon et al., "Can Work Make You Sick?"

22. Jay Kandiah, Melissa Yake, and Heather Willett, "Effects of Stress on Eating Practices among Adults," *Family and Consumer Sciences Research Journal* 37, no. 1 (September 2008): 27–38.

23. Ibid.

24. J. Liu et al., "The Melanocortinergic Pathway Is Rapidly Recruited by Acute Emotional Stress and Contributes to Stress-Induced Anorexia and Anxiety-Like Behavior," *Endocrinology* 148, no. 11 (November 2007): 5531–40.

25. Masahiro Ochi et al., "Effect of Chronic Stress on Gastric Emptying and Plasma Ghrelin Levels in Rats," *Life Science* 82, no. 15–16 (April 9, 2008): 862–68.

26. Ricard Farré et al., "Critical Role of Stress in Increased Oesophageal Mucosa Permeability and Dilated Intercellular Spaces," *Gut* 56, no. 9 (February 2007): 1191–97.

27. Martin E. Keck and Florian Holsboer, "Hyperactivity of CRH Neuronal Circuits as a Target for Therapeutic Interventions in Affective Disorders," *Peptides* 22, no. 5 (May 2001): 835–44.

28. T. G. Pickering, "Blood Platelets, Stress, and Cardiovascular Disease," *Psychosomatic Medicine* 55, no. 6 (November/December 1993): 483–84; E. M. Sternberg, "Does Stress Make You Sick and Belief Make You Well? The Science Connecting Body and Mind," *Annals of the New York Academy of Sciences* 917 (January 2000): 1–3.

29. Bert Garssen, "Psychological Factors and Cancer Development: Evidence after 30 Years of Research," *Clinical Psychology Review* 24, no. 3 (July 2004): 315–38; Eric Raible and Allan S. Jaffe, "Work Stress May Be a Determinant of Coronary Heart Disease," *Cardiology Today* 11, no. 3 (March 2008): 33; S. O. Dalton et al., "Mind and Cancer: Do Psychological Factors Cause Cancer?" *European Journal of Cancer* 38, no. 10 (July 2002): 1313–23; Edna M. V. Reiche, Sandra O. V. Nunes, and Helena K. Morimoto, "Stress, Depression, the Immune System, and Cancer," *Lancet Oncology* 5, no. 10 (October 2004): 617–25; Ljudmila Stojanovich and Dragomir Marisavljevich, "Stress as a Trigger of Autoimmune Disease," *Autoimmunity Reviews* 7, no. 3 (January 2008): 209–13; Eva M. Selhub, "Stress and Distress in Clinical Practice: A Mind-Body Approach," *Nutrition and Clinical Care* 5, no. 4 (July/August 2002): 182–90.

30. Meredith Melnick, "Study: Your Hostile Workplace May Be Killing You," *Time.com*, August 10, 2011, http://healthland.time.com/2011/08/10/study-your-hostile-work-place-may-be-killing-you/.

31. P. Butterworth et al., "The Psychosocial Quality of Work Determines Whether Employment Has Benefits for Mental Health: Results from a Longitudinal National Household Panel Survey," *Occupational and Environmental Medicine* 68, no. 11 (2011): 806–12.

32. Robert Pear, "Gap in Life Expectancy Widens for the Nation," *New York Times*, March 23, 2008, http://www.nytimes.com/2008/03/23/us/23health.html.

33. A. Antonovsky, "Social Class, Life Expectancy, and Overall Mortality," *Milbank Memorial Fund Quarterly* 45, no. 2 (April 1967): 31–73; Raymond Illsley and Deborah Baker, "Contextual Variations in the Meaning of Health Inequality," *Social Science and Medicine* 32, no. 4 (1991): 359–65; Tom Reynolds, "Report Examines Association between Cancer and Socioeconomic Status," *Journal of the National Cancer Institute* 95, no. 19 (2003): 1431–33.

34. "Are Poor People Less Likely to Be Healthy than Rich People?" Public Health Agency of Canada, September 11, 2008.

35. "Rich People Die Differently," *WebMD*, July 7, 2005, http://men.webmd.com/news/20050707/rich-people-die-differently.

36. Dan Seligman, "Why the Rich Live Longer," *Forbes.com*, June 7, 2004, http://www
.forbes.com/forbes/2004/0607/113_print.html.

37. Graham S. Lowe, Grant Schellenberg, and Harry S. Shannon, "Correlates of Employees' Perceptions of a Healthy Work Environment," *American Journal of Health
Promotion* 17, no. 6 (July/August 2003): 390–99; Katherine Baicker, David Cutler, and
Zirui Song, "Workplace Wellness Programs Can Generate Savings," *Health Affairs* 29,
no. 2 (February 2010): 304–11.

38. Beata Tobiasz-Adamczyk and Piotr Brzyski, "Psychosocial Work Conditions as
Predictors of Quality of Life at the Beginning of Older Age," *International Journal of
Occupational Medicine and Environmental Health* 18, no. 1 (January 2005): 43–52; T.
Theorell, "Working Conditions and Health," in *Social Epidemiology*, ed. L. F. Berkman
and I. Kawachi (New York: Oxford University Press, 2000), 95–117; E. B. Faragher,
M. Cass, and C. L. Cooper, "The Relationship between Job Satisfaction and Health:
A Meta-Analysis," *Occupational and Environmental Medicine* 62, no. 2 (February 2005):
105–12; R. Veenhoven, "Healthy Happiness: Effects of Happiness on Physical Health
and the Consequences for Preventive Health Care," *Journal of Happiness Studies*
9, no. 3 (September 2008): 449–69; Justina A. V. Fischer and Alfonso Sousa-Poza,
"Does Job Satisfaction Improve the Health of Workers? New Evidence Using Panel
Data and Objective Measures of Health," *Health Economics* 18, no. 1 (January 2009):
71–89.

39. Joachim C. Brunstein, "Personal Goals and Subjective Well-Being: A Longitudinal Study," *Journal of Personality and Social Psychology* 65, no. 5 (November 1993):
1061–70.

40. Nancy Cantor, "From Thought to Behavior: 'Having' and 'Doing' in the Study of
Personality and Cognition," *American Psychologist* 45, no. 6 (June 1990): 735–50.

41. Amanda Enayati, "A Creative Life Is a Healthy Life," *CNN.com*, May 26, 2012, http://
www.cnn.com/2012/05/25/health/enayati-innovation-passion-stress/index.html.

42. Marti Hand, "The Benefits of Integrating Creativity in Healthcare," Creativity in
Healthcare, accessed May 15, 2012, http://creativityinhealthcare.com/creativity
-in-healthcaremarti-handarts-in-healthcarehealthcarenursing-3/; Gene D. Cohen
et al., "The Impact of Professionally Conducted Cultural Programs on the Physical
Health, Mental Health, and Social Functioning of Older Adults," *Gerontologist* 46,
no. 6 (2006): 726–34; Daniel A. Monti et al., "A Randomized, Controlled Trial of
Mindfulness-Based Art Therapy (MBAT) for Women with Cancer," *Psychooncology* 15,
no. 5 (May 2006): 363–73; Bonnie Gabriel et al., "Art Therapy with Adult Bone Marrow Transplant Patients in Isolation: A Pilot Study," *Psychooncology* 10, no. 2 (March/
April 2001): 114–13; Joe Verghese et al., "Leisure Activities and the Risk of Demen-
tia in the Elderly," *New England Journal of Medicine* 348 (June 2003): 2508–16; R. F.
Cruz and D. L. Sabers, "Dance/Movement Therapy Is More Effective than Previously
Reported," *The Arts in Psychotherapy* 25 (1998): 101–104.

Chapter 7

1. Ruut Veenhoven, "World Database of Happiness: Continuous Register of Research
on Subjective Appreciation of Life," in *Challenges for Quality of Life in the Contemporary World: Advances in Quality-of-Life Studies, Theory and Research*, ed. W. Glatzer,

S. von Below, and M. Stoffregen (Dordrecht, The Netherlands: Kluwer Academic Publishers, 2004).

2. Corey L. M. Keyes, "Mental Illness and/or Mental Health? Investigating Axioms of the Complete State Model of Health," *Journal of Consulting and Clinical Psychology* 73, no. 3 (Jun 2005): 539–48.

3. Thomson Healthcare, Washington, D.C. "Ranking America's Mental Health: An Analysis of Depression across the States," *Mental Health America*, December 11, 2007, http://www.mentalhealthamerica.net/go/state-ranking.

4. National Institute of Mental Health, "Any Mood Disorder Among Adults," accessed May 15, 2012, http://www.nimh.nih.gov/statistics/1ANYMOODDIS_ADULT.shtml.

5. R. Veenhoven, *Conditions of Happiness* (Dordrecht, The Netherlands: Kluwer Academic Publishers, 1984).

6. Lawrence LeShan, "Cancer Mortality Rate: Some Statistical Evidence of the Effect of Psychological Factors," *Archives of General Psychiatry* 6, no. 5 (May 1962): 333–35; Reiner Rugulies, "Depression as a Predictor for Coronary Heart Disease: A Review and Meta-Analysis," *American Journal of Preventive Medicine* 23, no. 1 (July 2002): 51–61; Redford B. Williams and Neil Schneiderman, "Resolved: Psychosocial Interventions Can Improve Clinical Outcomes in Organic Disease," *Psychosomatic Medicine* 64, no. 4 (July/August 2002): 552–57; Robert Anda et al., "Depressed Affect, Hopelessness, and the Risk of Ischemic Heart Disease in a Cohort of US adults," *Epidemiology* 4, no. 4 (July 1993): 285–94; Anne Harrington, *The Placebo Effect: An Interdisciplinary Exploration* (Cambridge, MA: Harvard University Press, 1999), 60; Biing-Jiun Shen et al., "Anxiety Characteristics Independently and Prospectively Predict Myocardial Infarction in Men: The Unique Contribution of Anxiety among Psychological Factors," *Journal of the American College of Cardiology* 51, no. 2 (January 2008): 113–19; R. M. Gallagher and S. Cariati, "The Pain-Depression Conundrum: Bridging the Body and Mind," *Medscape Today Clinical Update*, October 2, 2002; D. C. Turk, "Beyond the Symptoms: The Painful Manifestations of Depression" (paper presented at Pain and Depression: Navigating the Intersection of Body and Mind Symposium, San Diego, August 20, 2002).

7. P. McCarron et al., "Temperament in Young Adulthood and Later Mortality: Prospective Observational Study," *Journal of Epidemiology and Community Health* 57, no. 11 (November 2003): 888–92; LeShan, "Cancer Mortality Rate: Some Statistical Evidence of the Effect of Psychological Factors"; Sabrina Paterniti et al., "Sustained Anxiety and 4-Year Progression of Carotid Atherosclerosis," *Arteriosclerosis, Thrombosis, and Vascular Biology* 21 (2001): 136–41.

8. Ed Diener and Micaela Chan, "Happy People Live Longer: Subjective Well-Being Contributes to Health and Longevity," *Applied Psychology: Health and Well-Being* 3, no. 1 (March 2011): 1–43.

9. Ibid.

10. Yoichi Chida and Andrew Steptoe. "Positive Psychological Well-Being and Mortality: A Quantitative Review of Prospective Observational Studies," *Psychosomatic Medicine* 70, no. 7 (September 2008): 741–56.

11. Michael Lemonick, "The Biology of Joy," *Time,* January 9, 2005.

12. Joshua Wolf Shenk, "What Makes Us Happy?" *Atlantic,* January 2009, http://www
    .theatlantic.com/magazine/archive/2009/06/what–makes–us–happy/7439/#.

13. Bernie S. Siegel, *Love, Medicine & Miracles* (New York: Harper & Row, 1986), 76.

14. Christopher Peterson, Martin E. Seligman, and George E. Vaillant, "Pessimistic Ex-
    planatory Style Is a Risk Factor for Physical Illness: A Thirty-Five-Year Longitudinal
    Study," *Journal of Personality and Social Psychology* 55, no. 1 (July 1988): 23–27.

15. Lisa G. Aspinwall and Richard G. Tedeschi, "The Value of Positive Psychology for
    Health Psychology: Progress and Pitfalls in Examining the Relation of Positive Phe-
    nomena to Health," *Annals of Behavioral Medicine* 39, no. 1 (February 2010): 4–15.

16. Erik J. Giltay et al., "Dispositional Optimism and All-Cause and Cardiovascular
    Mortality in a Prospective Cohort of Elderly Dutch Men and Women," *Archives of
    General Psychiatry* 61, no. 11 (November 2004): 1126–35.

17. Sheldon Cohen et al., "Positive Emotional Style Predicts Resistance to Illness after
    Experimental Exposure to Rhinovirus or Influenza A Virus," *Psychosomatic Medicine*
    68, no. 6 (November 1, 2006): 809–15.

18. Lemonick, "The Biology of Joy."

19. Martin Seligman, *Learned Optimism: How to Change Your Mind and Your Life* (New
    York: Vintage Books, 1991).

20. Christopher Peterson and Mechele E. De Avila, "Optimistic Explanatory Style and
    the Perception of Health Problems," *Journal of Clinical Psychology* 51, no. 1 (Janu-
    ary 1995): 128–32; Kymberley K. Bennett and Marta Elliott, "Pessimistic Explana-
    tory Style and Cardiac Health: What Is the Relation and the Mechanism that Links
    Them?" *Basic and Applied Social Psychology* 27, no. 3 (September 2005): 239–48; Katri
    Räikkönen et al., "Effects of Optimism, Pessimism, and Trait Anxiety on Ambula-
    tory Blood Pressure and Mood During Everyday Life," *Journal of Personality and Social
    Psychology* 76, no. 1 (January 1999): 104–13.

21. Christopher Peterson, "Explanatory Style as a Risk Factor for Illness," *Cognitive
    Therapy and Research* 12, no. 2 (1988): 119–32.

22. Laura D. Kubzansky and Rebecca C. Thurston, "Emotional Vitality and Incident
    Coronary Heart Disease: Benefits of Healthy Psychological Functioning," *Archives of
    General Psychiatry* 64, no. 12 (December 2007): 1393–1401.

23. Shelley E. Taylor et al., "Are Self-Enhancing Cognitions Associated with Healthy or
    Unhealthy Biological Profiles?" *Journal of Personality and Social Psychology* 85, no. 4
    (October 2003): 605–15.

24. Christopher Peterson and Martin E. Seligman, "Causal Explanations as a Risk Factor
    for Depression: Theory and Evidence," *Psychological Review* 91 no. 3 (July 1984):
    347–74.

25. Chida and Steptoe, "Positive Psychological Well-Being and Mortality."

26. M. A. Visintainer, J. R. Volpicelli, and M. E. Seligman, "Tumor Rejection in Rats after
    Inescapable or Escapable Shock," *Science* 216, no. 4544 (April 23, 1982): 437–39.

27. M. Seligman and M. Visintainer, "Tumor Rejection and Early Experience of Un-
    controllable Shock in the Rat," in *Affect, Conditioning, and Cognition: Essays on the*

Determinants of Behavior, ed. F. R. Brush and J. B. Overmier (Hillsdale, NJ: Erlbaum, 1985), 203–5.

28. Ellen J. Langer and Judith Rodin, "Effects of Choice and Enhanced Personal Responsibility for the Aged: A Field Experiment in an Institutional Setting," *Journal of Personality and Social Psychology* 34, no. 2 (1976): 191–98.

29. Martin Seligman, *Authentic Happiness: Using the New Positive Psychology to Realize Your Potential for Lasting Fulfillment* (New York: Free Press, 2003).

30. Deborah D. Danner, David A. Snowdon, and Wallace V. Friesen, "Positive Emotions in Early Life and Longevity: Findings from the Nun Study," *Journal of Personality and Social Psychology* 80, no. 5 (May 2001): 804–13.

31. R. Veenhoven, "Healthy Happiness: Effects of Happiness on Physical Health and the Consequences for Preventive Health Care," *Journal of Happiness Studies* 9, no. 3 (September 2008): 449–69.

32. Janice K. Kiecolt-Glaser et al., "Hostile Marital Interactions, Proinflammatory Cytokine Production, and Wound Healing," *Archives of General Psychiatry* 62, no. 12 (December 2005): 1377–84; Janice K. Kiecolt-Glaser et al., "Emotions, Morbidity, and Mortality: New Perspectives from Psychoneuroimmunology," *Annual Review of Psychology* 53 (February 2002): 83–107.

33. J. Licinio, P. W. Gold, and M. L. Wong, "A Molecular Mechanism for Stress-Induced Alterations in Susceptibility to Disease," *Lancet* 346, no. 8967 (July 1995): 104–6; Ryan T. Howell, Margaret L. Kern, and Sonja Lyubomirsky, "Health Benefits: Meta-Analytically Determining the Impact of Well-Being on Objective Health Outcomes," *Health Psychology Review* 1, no. 1 (July 2007): 83–136.

34. Lemonick, "The Biology of Joy"; Erin S. Costanzo et al., "Mood and Cytokine Response to Influenza Virus in Older Adults," *Journals of Gerontology* 59, no. 12 (December 2004): 1328–33; Marian L. Kohut et al., "Exercise and Psychosocial Factors Modulate Immunity to Influenza Vaccine in Elderly Individuals," *Journals of Gerontology* 57, no. 9 (September 2002): 557–62.

35. R. W. Bartrop et al., "Depressed Lymphocyte Function after Bereavement," *Lancet* 1, no. 8016 (April 16, 1977): 834–36.

36. D. M. Byrnes et al., "Stressful Events, Pessimism, Natural Killer Cell Cytotoxicity, and Cytotoxic/Suppressor T Cells in HIV+ Black Women at Risk for Cervical Cancer," *Psychosomatic Medicine* 60, no. 6 (November/December 1998): 714–22.

37. Peter Kirsch et al., "Oxytocin Modulates Neural Circuitry for Social Cognition and Fear in Humans," *Journal of Neuroscience* 25, no. 49 (December 7, 2005): 11489–93; C. Sue Carter, "Neuroendocrine Perspectives on Social Attachment and Love," *Psychoneuroendocrinology* 23, no. 8 (November 1998): 779–818.

38. Tiina-Mari Lyyra, "Predictors of Mortality in Old Age: Contribution of Self-Rated Health, Physical Functions, Life Satisfaction and Social Support on Survival among Older People," *University of Jyväskylä: Studies in Sport, Physical Education and Health* 119 (2006).

39. Diener and Chan, "Happy People Live Longer"; Lemonick, "The Biology of Joy"; Chida and Steptoe, "Positive Psychological Well-Being and Mortality."

40. S. Levy et al., "Survival Hazards Analysis in First Recurrent Breast Cancer Patients: Seven Year Follow Up," *Psychosomatic Medicine* 50, no. 5 (September/October 1988): 520–28.

41. Veenhoven, "Healthy Happiness"; Leonard R. Derogatis, Martin D. Abeloff, and Nick Melisaratos, "Psychological Coping Mechanisms and Survival Time in Metastatic Breast Cancer," *Journal of the American Medical Association* 242, no. 14 (October 5, 1979): 1504–8.

42. Frits Van Dam, "Does Happiness Heal," in *How Harmful Is Happiness? Consequences of Enjoying Life or Not,* ed. R. Veenhoven (The Netherlands: Universitaire Pers Rotterdam, 1989), 17–23.

43. Richard E. Lucas et al., "Reexamining Adaptation and the Set Point Model of Happiness: Reactions to Changes in Marital Status," *Journal of Personality and Social Psychology* 84, no. 3 (March 2003): 527–39.

44. Sonja Lyubomirsky, Kennon M. Sheldon, and David Schkade, "Pursuing Happiness: The Architecture of Sustainable Change," *Review of General Psychology* 9, no. 2 (June 2005): 111–31.

45. S. W. Cole et al., "Accelerated Course of Human Immunodeficiency Virus Infection in Gay Men Who Conceal Their Homosexual Identity," *Psychosomatic Medicine* 58, no. 3 (May/June 1996): 219–31.

Chapter 8

1. "Easy Ways to Take the Edge Off," *ABC News Video,* April 22, 2009, http://abcnews .go.com/video/playerIndex?id=7392433.

2. "Eliciting the Relaxation Response," Benson-Henry Institute for Mind Body Medicine, Massachusetts General Hospital, accessed May 15, 2012, http://www .massgeneral.org/bhi/basics/eliciting_rr.aspx.

3. Richard J. Davidson et al., "Alterations in Brain and Immune Function Produced by Mindfulness Meditation," *Psychosomatic Medicine* 65, no. 4 (July/August 2003): 564–70.

4. Bonnie Horrigan, "Meditation Reduces Pain Scores," *Explore: The Journal of Science and Healing* 7, no. 4 (July/August 2011): 215–16; R. Manocha et al., "A Randomized, Controlled Trial of Meditation for Work Stress, Anxiety and Depressed Mood in Full-Time Workers,". *Evidence-Based Complementary and Alternative Medicine* (June 7, 2011); W. P. Smith, W. C. Compton, and W. B. West, "Meditation as an Adjunct to a Happiness Enhancement Program," *Journal of Clinical Psychology* 51, no. 2 (March 1995): 269–73; A. Nesvold et al., "Increased Heart Rate Variability during Nondirective Meditation," *European Journal of Preventive Cardiology* 19, no. 4 (August 2012): 773–80; F. Zeidan et al., "Mindfulness Meditation Improves Cognition: Evidence of Brief Mental Training," *Consciousness and Cognition 19,* no. 2 (June 10, 2010): 597–605; L. Fortney and M. Taylor, "Meditation in Medical Practice: A Review of the Evidence and Practice," *Primary Care* 37, no. 1 (March 2010): 81–90; R. Walsh and S. L. Shapiro, "The Meeting of Meditative Disciplines and Western Psychology: A Mutually Enriching Dialogue," *American Psychologist* 61, no. 3 (April 2006): 227–39; Maura Paul-Labrador et al., "Effects of a Randomized Controlled Trial of Transcen-

dental Meditation on Components of the Metabolic Syndrome in Subjects with Coronary Heart Disease," *Archives of Internal Medicine* 166, no. 11 (June 12, 2006): 1218–24; S. I. Nidich et al., "A Randomized Controlled Trial of the Effects of Transcendental Meditation on Quality of Life in Older Breast Cancer Patients," *Integrative Cancer Therapy* 8, no. 3 (September 2009): 228–34.

5.   F. Zeidan et al., "Effects of Brief and Sham Mindfulness Meditation on Mood and Cardiovascular Variables," *Alternative and Complementary Medicine* 16, no. 8 (August 2010): 867–73.

6.   Ann MacDonald, "Using the Relaxation Response to Reduce Stress," *Harvard Health Publications,* November 10, 2010, http://www.health.harvard.edu/blog/using-the -relaxation-response-to-reduce-stress-20101110780.

7.   Jeffery A. Dusek et al., "Genomic Counter-Stress Changes Induced by the Relaxation Response," *PLoS ONE* 3, no. 7 (July 2008).

8.   "Almost a Quarter of All Disease Caused by Environmental Exposure," World Health Organization, June 16, 2006, http://www.who.int/mediacentre/news/releases/2006 /pr32/en/index.html.

Chapter 9

1.   Kelly Ann Turner. "Spontaneous Remission of Cancer: Theories from Healers, Physicians, and Cancer Survivors," Fall 2010, http://www.shuniyahealing.com/offer /research.html.

ACKNOWLEDGMENTS

Writing a book is like giving birth. You might have to go through labor and do the pushing, but it takes a whole team of midwives to support you through the gestation and usher your baby out into the world. I have been blessed with dozens of midwives, and to those who supported my process, I am infinitely grateful.

Ginormous thanks to my agent, Michele Martin, who invited me to write the one book I could spend the rest of my life shouting from the rooftops. There will be many more books, but that one invitation changed everything for me. I seriously adore you and am overflowing with gratitude for how far above and beyond you went, supporting me through this book. I feel so lucky you came into my life right when this book was ready to come through me.

To Reid Tracy, Louise Hay, Patty Gift, Sally Mason, and the rest of the team at Hay House, thank you for seeing my diamond in the rough, allowing me to wander through the labyrinth as I honed in on my message, and inviting me into the family. I still pinch myself. Often. I feel blessed.

To my husband and tireless research assistant, Matt Klein, bless you, my love. You know researching and writing this book was a Herculean task, and I couldn't have done it without your support, love, childcare assistance, sushi wraps, and kisses. I am the luckiest woman in the world to wake up next to you every day.

To Siena Klein, thank you for still loving me, even when I was burning the midnight oil, researching and writing this book when you wanted me to color with you in your Hello Kitty coloring books. When I asked you if you were mad at me for working so hard and you said, "Mommy, I understand the world needs you," you healed me. I have the most precious daughter ever, and I promise there will be roller coasters when this is all over!

To Melanie Bates, OwningPink.com's editor, my assistant, my unofficial therapist, and my beloved friend, thank you for being the daily sounding board for the ideas that bubbled up as I researched and wrote this book. Transmuting fuzzy thoughts into language people can understand is no small task, but you made it feel like a picnic. I loved learning all this with you by my side, and I will always consider this book part yours. You once told me it was part of your calling to help me bring my message into the world, and darling—phew! We've done it. Thank you.

A huge thank you to Tricia Barrett, for helping me compose the questions in the Diagnostic Exercise #3 in the Make The Diagnosis for Yourself section of the last chapter. Your intuitive gifts and ability to tap into collective consciousness made that section so much richer. Thank you also for holding my soul in your heart as I learned my lessons and for making me believe that anything is possible when it comes to health. Your support, wisdom, counseling, and accountability made this book—and me—all the better. Plus, you're a bushel of fun, I love your laugh, you look hot in those pants you borrowed, and I just adore you!

To the pioneers whose work inspired me and whose research made mine easier: Rachel Naomi Remen, Christiane Northrup, Bernie Siegel, Larry Dossey, Dean Ornish, Andrew Weil, Anne Harrington, Ted Kaptchuk, Bruce Lipton, Fabrizio Benedetti, Norman Cousins, Joan Borysenko, Deepak Chopra, Frank Lipman, Mehmet Oz, Mark Hyman, Herbert Benson, Arnold A. Hutschnecker, Louise Hay, Martin Seligman, Sonja Lyubomirsky, Brené Brown—thank you for blazing the trail so I could skip-to-my-lou along a well-worn trail until I hit the path I had to blaze on my own. I'm infinitely grateful to you all for all you've done to contribute to the mind-body medicine movement that is on its way to becoming mainstream because of you.

A giant thank you to Marilyn Schlitz, Cassandra Vieten, Caryle Hirshberg, Brendan O'Regan, and all the people at the Institute of Noetic Sciences for all the work you put into studying how the mind can heal the body. Your Spontaneous Remission Project was a godsend, and your friendship and professional support is SO appreciated.

A huge thank you to Kris Carr, who, as promised, "gives great foreword." Thank you for being such an inspiration, for boldly demonstrating that anyone facing an illness can use it as an opportunity to awaken, for teaching people about using food as preventive medicine and disease treatment, for your mentorship and guidance, for being my shero, and most importantly, for your precious friendship. I cherish you.

To my mother, Trish Rankin, thank you for listening as I prattled on about what I was learning, and for holding space for me to evolve, even when the choices I was making and the views I was expressing were a radical leap from what Dad and everyone in medical school taught me to believe. When people experience a radical life shift, often they lose those they love most. But you, you're the best mother in the world. I have always known I had your blessing to fly toward whatever North Star called me to it. Thank you for loving and accepting me, for being proud of me, even when I'm pushing the envelope. I love you.

A very special, resounding, roof-shouting thanks to my mastermind group of rock-star authors and speakers: Amy Ahlers, Christine Arylo, Mike Robbins, and Steve Sisgold. Not only have each of you touched my life and my heart in immeasurable ways; you've also made this book possible. Thank you for your professional and spiritual guidance as I bumbled my way along this path and finally found my way. Having you in my life makes its way into my gratitude journal almost every single day. I love you all so much.

Thank you, Elisabeth Manning, for spiritual guidance, inspiration, tools for tapping in, friendship, and being a frequent sounding board. You are a blessing. Thank you, Dana Theus, for many rousing discussions about whole health, for guidance from angels, for mentoring on my often-misguided leadership efforts, and for a friendship I cherish. Thank you, Cari Hernandez, for serving as a sounding board and bearing witness to this journey with love, tea, and the best kind of friendship. Thank you, Nicholas Wilton, for fueling my creative fire and teaching me what an overflowing jar of marbles feels like.

I feel so much gratitude for all the mentors and teachers who played a huge part in my personal and professional journey. Thank you especially to Debbie Rosas, Sheila Kelley, Barbara Stanny, SARK, Regena Thomashauer, Anne Davin, Danielle LaPorte, Chris Guillebeau, Jonathan Fields, Tama Kieves, Frank Lipman, and Brené Brown. You and your teachings saved me from myself, and I will always be eternally grateful.

A huge thank you to Martha Beck, who modeled what it means to be brave and helped me find my North Star years ago, and more recently, who made me realize I'm no longer a lonely little puddle but part of an ocean of wayfinders and menders collectively raising the vibration of the planet. I love you wordlessly and am so grateful for your friendship.

Thank you to Fred Kraziese, Bob Uslander, and Ken Jaques for being the health-care revolutionaries nudging me to make the call to action necessary in order to bring a new kind of medicine into the world in a bigger way.

Thank you to Rachel Carlton Abrams, Joanne Perron, Aviva Romm, and Kim Goodwin for letting me pick your doctor brains, offering me vital feedback, and giving me so much hope for the future of medicine.

Thank you to Kate McPhail for encouraging me to write this book as if I were giving expert testimony in front of a jury of my peers (and for being such a beloved friend).

Thank you to Rob Zeps, for being my favorite skeptic.

Thank you to Barbara Poelle (a.k.a. "Monkey Barbara") for being willing to get in a monkey knife fight to help me bring my message to the world, for believing in me when nobody else did, and for setting me free with love when it was time to fly.

Thank you to everyone at Clear Center of Health, especially Dr. Beth McDougall, for teaching me so much, for giving me the opportunity to practice medicine the way I always believed it was possible, for giving me the chance to learn what I needed to learn, and for setting me free when it was time for me to move on. I'll always be grateful for the precious time I spent with you and the healing you offered me after medicine left me more than a little wounded.

Thank you to Lisa Brent, Colin Smikle, Lakenda Wallace, and Susan Fox for helping me give birth to the Owning Pink Center, where I learned and practiced so many of the lessons I share in this book. I'm eternally grateful to each of you.

Thank you to Joy Mazzola, Lauren Nagel, and Megan Monique Lewis for putting up with me when I was so busy learning and not quite ready to teach or lead. I appreciate all you did.

Thank you to Katsy Johnson, Chris, Keli, Kim, Malen, Nick, Trudy, and Larry Rankin, Izayah Graham, Rebecca Bass Ching, the Wirick clan, April Sweazy, Genevieve Leck, Diane Zeps, Kandy Lozano, Vera Sparre, Scott Richards, Maya and Jochen Pechak, Geoff Rogers, Lawrence Kolin, Stephanie Walker, Tori Mordecai, Jory Des Jardins, and Kira Siebert—just because I love you.

And finally, but very importantly, a huge thank you to everyone in the OwningPink.com and LissaRankin.com communities, to those who follow me on Twitter at @lissarankin, to my Facebook friends, to those who read and comment on my newsletters, and to those who subscribe to the Daily Flame. You all held such beautiful space and provided such critical feedback as I navigated the journey of this book. You have no idea how your posts, comments, e-mails, and tweets shaped what I wrote in this book. I am eternally grateful for you. You are why I wrote this book.

ABOUT THE AUTHOR

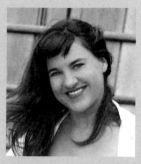 **Lissa Rankin MD** is a physician, coach for visionaries and healers, author, speaker, artist, blogger and founder of the online health and wellness communities OwningPink.com and LissaRankin.com. Lissa is committed to helping people heal, connect and thrive, not just in their bodies but in their hearts and souls. She is also passionate about supporting other visionaries, healers and coaches who share her desire to help others become wholly healthy in all aspects of their lives. When not travelling the world spreading her message, Lissa loves painting in her encaustic studio, skiing in Lake Tahoe, practising yoga, dancing and hiking near the ocean and among the redwoods in Marin County, California, where she lives with her husband, Matt, her daughter, Siena and her dog, Bezoar. Follow her blog to read 'Passionate Prescriptions for Living and Loving Fearlessly'.

www.owningpink.com
www.lissarankin.com

HAY HOUSE TITLES OF RELATED INTEREST

YOU CAN HEAL YOUR LIFE, the movie, starring Louise L. Hay & Friends
(available as a 1-DVD programme and an expanded 2-DVD set)
Watch the trailer at: **www.LouiseHayMovie.com**

THE SHIFT, the movie, starring Dr Wayne W. Dyer
(available as a 1-DVD programme and an expanded 2-DVD set)
Watch the trailer at: **www.DyerMovie.com**

———————

ALL IS WELL: Heal Your Body with Medicine, Affirmations, and Intuition,
by Louise L. Hay and Mona Lisa Schulz, MD

*THE BIOLOGY OF BELIEF: Unleashing the Power of Consciousness, Matter,
and Miracles,* by Bruce H. Lipton, PhD

*CRAZY SEXY KITCHEN: 150 Plant-Empowered Recipes to
Ignite a Mouthwatering Revolution,* by Kris Carr

HOW YOUR MIND CAN HEAL YOUR BODY,
by David R. Hamilton, PhD

REVEAL: A Sacred Manual for Getting Spiritually Naked,
by Meggan Watterson

THE TAPPING SOLUTION: A Revolutionary System for Stress-Free Living,
by Nick Ortner

All of the above are available at your local bookstore,
or may be ordered by contacting Hay House (see next page).

———————

We hope you enjoyed this Hay House book. If you'd like to receive our online catalogue featuring additional information on Hay House books and products, or if you'd like to find out more about the Hay Foundation, please contact:

Hay House UK, Ltd., Astley House, 33 Notting Hill Gate, W11 3JQ
Phone: 0-20-3675-2450 • *Fax:* 0-20-3675-2451
www.hayhouse.co.uk • **www.hayfoundation.org**

Published and distributed in the United States by: Hay House, Inc., P.O. Box 5100, Carlsbad, CA 92018-5100 • *Phone:* (760) 431-7695 or (800) 654-5126
Fax: (760) 431-6948 or (800) 650-5115
www.hayhouse.com®

Published and distributed in Australia by: Hay House Australia Pty. Ltd., 18/36 Ralph St., Alexandria NSW 2015 • *Phone:* 612-9669-4299 • *Fax:* 612-9669-4144
www.hayhouse.com.au

Published and distributed in the Republic of South Africa by: Hay House SA (Pty), Ltd., P.O. Box 990, Witkoppen 2068 • *Phone/Fax:* 27-11-467-8904 • www.hayhouse.co.za

Published in India by: Hay House Publishers India, Muskaan Complex, Plot No. 3, B-2, Vasant Kunj, New Delhi 110 070 • *Phone:* 91-11-4176-1620 • *Fax:* 91-11-4176-1630
www.hayhouse.co.in

Distributed in Canada by: Raincoast, 9050 Shaughnessy St., Vancouver, B.C. V6P 6E5
Phone: (604) 323-7100 • *Fax:* (604) 323-2600 • www.raincoast.com

---

Take Your Soul on a Vacation

Visit **www.HealYourLife.com®** to regroup, recharge, and reconnect with your own magnificence. Featuring blogs, mind-body-spirit news, and life-changing wisdom from Louise Hay and friends.

Visit **www.HealYourLife.com** today!

JOIN THE HAY HOUSE FAMILY

As the leading self-help, mind, body and spirit publisher in the UK, we'd like to welcome you to our family so that you can enjoy all the benefits our website has to offer.

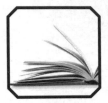 **EXTRACTS** from a selection of your favourite author titles

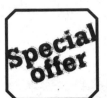 **COMPETITIONS, PRIZES & SPECIAL OFFERS** Win extracts, money off, downloads and so much more

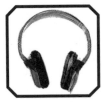 **LISTEN** to a range of radio interviews and our latest audio publications

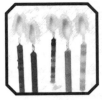 **CELEBRATE YOUR BIRTHDAY** An inspiring gift will be sent your way

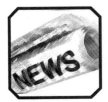 **LATEST NEWS** Keep up with the latest news from and about our authors

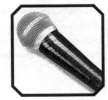 **ATTEND OUR AUTHOR EVENTS** Be the first to hear about our author events

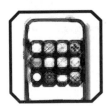 **iPHONE APPS** Download your favourite app for your iPhone

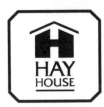 **HAY HOUSE INFORMATION** Ask us anything, all enquiries answered

join us online at **www.hayhouse.co.uk**

Astley House, 33 Notting Hill Gate
London W11 3JQ
T: 020 3675 2450 E: info@hayhouse.co.uk